LIM 18

SYNTHESIS OF PSYCHIATRIC CASES

WITHDRAWN 19/06/24.

Distributed worldwide by
Oxford University Press

Typeset by
Saxon Graphics Ltd., Derby

Printed in Great Britain by
Alden Press

SYNTHESIS OF PSYCHIATRIC CASES

Dr Vivienne Schnieden
MA (Cantab) MB BS MRCPsych FRANZCP

Consultant Liaison Psychiatrist
Director of Training
Prince of Wales Hospital
Sydney, Australia

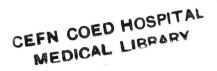

ACKNOWLEDGEMENTS

To my teachers in particular David Sturgeon, Gavin Andrews and Gordon Parker for their encouragement. To my colleagues Marie-Paule Austin, Lisa Lampe, Maryanne O'Donnell, Jan Russell, James Bell, Henry Brodaty, Philip Mitchell, Stella Engel, Angelo Virgona and Perminder Sachdev for their helpful comments.

To Greenwich Medical Media and Peter Sullivan for their support.

To the **American Psychiatric Association** for permission to adapt diagnostic criteria from the *Diagnostic and Statistical Manual of Mental Disorders*, Fourth Edition. Washington, DC, American Psychiatric Association, 1994.

To the authors of the following publications for permission to adapt material for use in this book:

Bird & Harrison. *Examination Notes in Psychiatry*, Second Edition, 1987. Wright, Bristol, UK.

ECDEU Assessment Manual for Psychopharmacology. 534–535 Guy W, US Department of Health, Education and Welfare (AIMS Scale).

Flaherty. *Psychiatry:Diagnosis and Treatment*, Second Edition. Appleton and Lange. Simon and Schuster International and Business & Professional Group. Stamford, CT, USA.

Guthrie & Creed *Seminars in Liaison Psychiatry*. Gaskell, 1996. Royal College of Psychiatrists 17 Belgrave Square, London, UK.

Kaplan & Sadock's *Synopsis of Psychiatry*. Williams & Wilkins. 351 West Camden Street, Baltimore, MD, USA.

Pierce Suicide Intent Score:*British Journal of Psychiatry* 1977; **130:** 377–385 Royal College of Psychiatrists, 17 Belgrave Square, London, UK.

Therapeutic Guidelines Limited. Level 3, 55 Flemington Road, North Melbourne, Victoria 3051, Australia.

Wells, C. E. Pseudodementia. *American Journal of Psychiatry* 1979; **136:** 898.

To my father

CONTENTS

INTRODUCTION

This book aims to provide trainees in psychiatry with a logical approach to clinical cases encountered in the postgraduate clinical examination. It illustrates some common and hypothetical cases and provides examples of possible areas examiners may explore which are relevant to these cases. This examination is designed to assess a candidate's clinical acumen and expertise. It is also a performance as the candidate has a limited time with the patient and also with the examiners in which to convince them that she or he is a competent and empathic clinician. The cases used are those most likely to be encountered in a clinical examination. They comprise disorders frequently encountered and illustrate some of the difficulties of diagnosis or management. Often candidates do themselves a disservice by concentrating on diagnostic possibilities and thereby omitting to emphasize the comorbidity and difficulties that this provides in the management of the case. The clinical examination aims to explore that the candidate is able to show an understanding of the patient seen and are able to formulate an appropriate management plan.

Candidates can prepare in a variety of ways, the most important being clinical work under supervision in their training scheme, and presenting to consultants and supervisors as a regular part of the training programme. Rehearsal in an unfamiliar setting with unknown examiners can also help to manage anxiety in the exam situation.

Managing anxiety is a large part of the exam process. It is also a necessary skill for a consultant who acts as leader of a multidisciplinary team. Candidates often disadvantage themselves by having inadequate control of their anxiety.

V.S.

Sydney

1998

AFFECTIVE DISORDERS

1.1 DEPRESSION

IDENTIFICATION

- Name, age, sex, culture, occupation, status (often isolated)
- Mean onset age 40 years, (50% have onset between ages 20 and 50 years) major depressive disorder

REFERRAL

Self, family, after deliberate self harm.

PRESENTING COMPLAINT

Symptoms of depression.
Use mnemonic *SIGE CAPS*

Sleep disturbed
Interest diminished
Guilt
Energy decreased
Concentration decreased
Appetite and weight up or down
Psychomotor retardation and agitation
Suicidal

HISTORY OF PRESENTING COMPLAINT

Any life events, losses, stress.

FAMILY HISTORY

- Genetics – increase in the first degree relatives of probands
- Adoption studies support genetic basis of mood disorder
- Increased depression, suicide, mania, alcohol in men (Winokur depressive spectrum)

PERSONAL HISTORY

- Neglect, abuse
- Learned helplessness
- Maternal loss before aged 11 years or poor relationship with primary carer

PAST MEDICAL HISTORY

Any serious illnesses or chronic condition.

PAST PSYCHIATRIC HISTORY

Any previous illnesses, treatment.

FORENSIC HISTORY

Nil.

PREMORBID PERSONALITY

Dependent, obsessive compulsive, hysterical.

MENTAL STATE EXAMINATION

- Stooped posture, hand wringing, hair pulling, no spontaneous movements, downcast averted gaze
- Mood, affect – depressed
- Talk – decreased rate
- Thought content – negative view of the world, self and others, suicidal ideation, death, poverty of content
- Delusions of guilt, worthlessness, nihilistic, poverty, mood congruent or incongruent, e.g. grandiose beliefs, persecutory beliefs
- Hallucinations – mood congruent, less complex than in schizophrenia
- Auditory hallucinations – second person, give short, clipped statements, e.g. 'you're worthless, kill yourself' rather than the running commentary experienced in schizophrenia
- Cognition – oriented to time, place and person
- Some impaired concentration and forgetfulness
- Impulse control – patients tend to be at risk of self harm when they start to improve and have energy needed to plan and carry out deliberate self harm
- Insight – often overemphasize symptoms and life problems

CRITERIA FOR MAJOR DEPRESSIVE EPISODE Modified with permission from the Diagnostic and Statistical Manual of Mental Disorders, Fourth Edition. Copyright 1994 American Psychiatric Association.

A. Five (or more) of the following features have been present during the same 2-week period and represent a change from previous functioning: at least one of the symptoms is either (1) depressed mood or (2) loss of interest or pleasure:

- Depressed mood most of the day, nearly every day as indicated by either subjective report (e.g. feels sad or empty) or observation made by others (e.g. appears tearful) (Note: in children or adolescents can be irritable mood)
- Markedly diminished interest or pleasure in all, or almost all activities most of the day, nearly everyday (as indicated by either subjective account or observation made by others)
- Significant weight loss when not dieting or weight gain (e.g. a change of >5% of body weight in a month), or decrease or increase in appetite nearly every day
- Insomnia or hypersomnia nearly every day
- Psychomotor agitation or retardation nearly every day (observable by others, not merely subjective feelings of restlessness or being slowed down)
- Fatigue or loss of energy nearly every day
- Feeling of worthlessness or excessive or inappropriate guilt (which may be delusional) nearly every day (not merely self-reproach or guilt about being sick)
- Diminished ability to think or concentrate or indecisiveness, nearly every day (either by subjective account or as observed by others)
- Recurrent thoughts of death (not just fear of dying), recurrent suicidal ideation without a specific plan, or a suicide attempt or a specific plan for committing suicide

B. Symptoms do not meet criteria for a mixed episode.

C. The symptoms cause clinically significant distress or impairment in social, occupational or other important areas of functioning.

D. The symptoms are not due to the direct physiological effects of a substance (e.g. drug of abuse, medication) or a general medical condition (e.g. hypothyroidism).

E. The symptoms are not better accounted for by Bereavement, i.e. after the loss of a loved one, the symptoms persist >2 months or are characterized by marked functional impairment, morbid preoccupation with worthlessness, suicidal ideation, psychotic symptoms or psychomotor retardation.

DIFFERENTIAL DIAGNOSIS

- Mood disorder due to a general medical condition*
- Substance-induced mood disorder – toxin, e.g. cocaine
- Dementia
- Manic episodes with irritable mood
- Mixed episodes – criteria met for both the major depressive episode and also manic episode
- Attention deficit disorder

- Adjustment disorder with depressed mood – full criteria not met for major depressive disorder
- Bereavement – persist for 2 months plus
- Periods of sadness
- Depressive disorder not otherwise specified

* General medical condition causing depression

- Central nervous system, Parkinson's, Huntington's, multiple sclerosis, cerebrovascular disease
- Encephalitis
- Metabolic – vitamin deficiencies, e.g. B_{12}, folate, pellagra
- Endocrine – diabetes, hypothyroidism, hyperadrenocorticism and hypoadrenocorticism
- Autoimmune conditions, e.g. systemic lupus erythematosis
- Viral, hepatitis, mononucleosis
- HIV
- Cancer, e.g. of the pancreas
- Tumours, e.g. of the frontal lobe
- Drugs, e.g. reserpine, propanolol, L-dopa, oral contraceptives, corticosteroids, alpha methyl dopa, amphetamine withdrawal, antipsychotic drugs

Current episode can be described as:

Psychotic or non psychotic
- Mood congruent delusions and hallucinations with depressive themes, e.g. personal inadequacy, guilt, disease, death, nihilism, deserved punishment
- Incongruent – e.g. persecutory delusions or thought insertion, possession and delusions of control

Mild, moderate, severe
- Mild, few symptoms in excess of those needed to make diagnosis
- Moderate – symptoms of functional impairment
- Severe – excess symptoms to make diagnosis and also a marked interference with social activities or relationships with others

CATATONIC FEATURES SPECIFIER   Modified with permission from the Diagnostic and Statistical Manual of Mental Disorders, Fourth Edition. Copyright 1994 American Psychiatric Association.

The clinical picture is dominated by at least two of the following:

- Motoric immobility as evidenced by catalepsy (including waxy flexibility) or stupor.
- Excessive motor activity (that is apparently purposeless and not influenced by external stimuli)
- Extreme negativism (an apparently motiveless resistance to all instructions or maintenance of a rigid posture against attempts to be moved) or mutism

- Peculiarities of voluntary movement as evidence by posturing (voluntary assumption of inappropriate or bizarre postures), stereotyped movements, prominent mannerisms or prominent grimacing
- Echolalia or echopraxia

DIFFERENTIAL DIAGNOSIS OF CATATONIC DISORDER

Catatonic disorder due to general medical condition, schizophrenia, catatonic type, side effect of medication, catatonic mood disorder mixed, manic, depressed, bipolar I or II.

MELANCHOLIC FEATURES SPECIFIER Modified with permission from the Diagnostic and Statistical Manual of Mental Disorders, Fourth Edition. Copyright 1994 American Psychiatric Association.

With melancholic features if:

A. Either of the following occur during the most severe period of the current episode:

- Loss of pleasure in all or almost all activities
- Lack of reactivity to usually pleasurable stimuli (does not feel much better even temporarily, when something good happens)

B. Three (or more) of the following:

- Distinct quality of depressed mood (i.e. the depressed mood is experienced as distinctly different from the kind of feeling experienced after the death of a loved one)
- Depression regularly worse in the morning
- Early morning awakening (at least 2 hours before usual time of awakening)
- Marked psychomotor retardation or agitation
- Significant anorexia or weight loss
- Excessive or inappropriate guilt

ATYPICAL FEATURES SPECIFIER Modified with permission from the Diagnostic and Statistical Manual of Mental Disorders, Fourth Edition. Copyright 1994 American Psychiatric Association.

With atypical features if:

A. Mood reactivity (i.e. mood brightens in response to actual or potential positive events).

B. Two (or more) of the following features:

- Significant weight gain or increase in appetite
- Hypersomnia
- Leaden paralysis (i.e. heavy, laden feelings in arms or legs)
- Long-standing pattern of interpersonal rejection sensitivity (not limited to episodes of mood disturbance) that results in significant social or occupational impairment

C. Criteria are not met for 'with melancholic features' or 'with catatonic features' during the same episode.

CRITERIA FOR POST PARTUM ONSET SPECIFIER Modified with permission from the Diagnostic and Statistical Manual of Mental Disorders, Fourth Edition. Copyright 1994 American Psychiatric Association.

With post partum onset – recent disorder within 4 weeks post partum

MANAGEMENT

Safety

- Inpatient or not – voluntary or not?
- Instructions to nursing staff

Clarify diagnosis

- Observations and disability – interactions with staff or on ward
- Exclude differential diagnosis

SPECIAL INVESTIGATIONS

To exclude ... I would do ...

FBC UE LFT TFT Ca, PO_4, glucose, B_{12}, folate, monospot urine – drug analysis.

- Collateral history from other source to verify information and to do what?
- Role of other professionals – to do what?

Establish a therapeutic alliance

Decrease symptoms using a biopsychosocial model

- Biological – SSRI, e.g. citalopram, sertraline, paroxitene, fluvoxamine, fluoxetine; SNRI, e.g. venlafaxine; Tricyclic, e.g. desipramine, nortryptiline, clomipramine, dothiepin; Heterocyclics, e.g. mianserin; RIMA, e.g. moclobemide; 5-HT antagonists, e.g. nefazadone
- Atypical depression – MAOIs, e.g. phenelazine – aim for 45-90 mg/day – start with 15 mg bd
- Adjunctive patient education that is accessible, user-friendly and culturally appropriate
- Social – support systems
- Occupational and recreational activities

LONG-TERM MANAGEMENT

- Untreated last 6–12 months up to 2 years; treated last 3 months
- Recurrences are common and 25% relapse in 6 months, 50% in 2 years and 50–75% in 5 years after ceasing treatment

Biological

- Maintenance therapy for 12–18 months after acute episode
- Prior to lithium – FBC, UE, TFT, Cr, pregnancy test, ECG
- Prior to ECT – FBC, blood profile, CXR, urine, ECG

Management of resistant depression

- Check history, diagnosis, compliance
- Exclude organic causes
- Check adequate administration of antidepressant (duration and dose)
- Exclude comorbid substance dependence
- Any personality, marital, psychosocial issues maintaining difficulties?
- Change to a different antidepressant class (including reversible MAOIs)
- Augment SSRI / SNRI / TCA with lithium, T_3 or pindolol (the latter for SSRIs only)
- Try ECT, two courses – one unilateral course then bilateral if not responsive
- Psychosurgery — patient's wish, other treatments fail, diagnosis appropriate and no contraindications

Electroconvulsive Therapy

- Main indications are for depression, mania, catatonic symptoms, unresponsive to antidepressants and actively suicidal
- Work up – review cardiac status, pulmonary status, endocrine functions, electrolytes.
- Treat two to three times a week
- Eight to 12 sessions
- Muscle relaxant – succinylcholine, barbiturate, anaesthesia
- Ventilate
- Supra-threshold dosing essential
- Seizure threshold increases with age and medications, male>female
- Unilateral, brief pulse
- Maintain on antidepressants after treatment
- Side effects – afterwards memory dysfunction
- Charge = voltage × current × time
- Withdraw medications prior to treatment such as benzodiazepines, anticonvulsants

Psychological

Insight oriented – ability to form alliance, relationship, insight.

Brief psychotherapy

Modify complaint, positive influence on patients adjustment and personality structure.

Supportive

Restore patient to level of functioning.

Cognitive Behavioural therapy

- Challenge unhelpful cognitions, assumptions
- Use diary, goal setting
- Lewinsohn's positive events schedule
- Depressed patients elicit fewer behaviours compared with controls
- Depressed patients have a lower rate of positive reinforcement compared with controls
- Increasing the number of pleasant activities affects mood
- More sensitive to aversive stimuli compared with non-depressed controls
- Increased rate of positive reinforcement occurs with clinical improvement

ENVIRONMENT

- Life events
- Social supports

Prognostic indicators

Depend on the duration of symptoms, psychosocial indicators of the course.

Poor prognosis

Dysthymia? Abuse of alcohol and other substances and a history of more than one depressive episode. Comorbid anxiety is common and may respond well to treatment (slow breathing technique, relaxation).

GRIEF

- Deal with losses and the cultural aspects of bereavement
- Grief work: withdraw attachment and work through pain of bereavement. Uncomplicated bereavement may experience shock, preoccupation with the deceased and resolution
- May decrease appetite, weight loss, dreams, survivor guilt, identification with the person

Anticipatory grief

Grieved loss in advance.

Pathological grief

Predisposing factors:
- Sudden horrible death
- Socially isolated
- Feel responsible
- Ambivalent relationship, unresolved conflict and dependent

Distinguish between grief and depression

- Grief is often intense, <2 months, no suicidal ideation, visions and voices of the deceased, pseudo-hallucinations, self-blame related to deceased, improvement over time
- Depression lasts longer, suicidal ideation is often present and sustained depressive delusions, pervasive depressed mood, focus on self, no change over time

During grief therapy ventilate appropriate sadness and anger, one-to-one therapy, self help, widow groups.

1.2 DEPRESSION CASE

IDENTIFICATION

82-year-old English woman, widowed, lives alone, voluntary patient.

ISSUES

Management of a patient with a depressive illness.

DIFFICULTIES

Hard to remember short-term events.

REFERRAL

Admitted 3 weeks ago on recommendation of psychiatrist.

PRESENTING COMPLAINT

- 'Gets depressed'
- Unable to cope with shopping or going out

HISTORY OF PRESENTING COMPLAINT

- Describes everything as an effort, gets upset by the slightest thing. Difficulty in sleeping and will wake up early in the morning, appetite poor, has lost weight (3 kg), energy poor, does not feel guilty, difficulty in concentrating, slowed movements, no suicidal ideation or intent
- Tearful and loss of enjoyment of anything (anhedonia)
- Symptoms have come on gradually in the past few months. Her family have become increasingly concerned about her and she has started to do things such as forgetting to pay bills unless she writes these things down
- No manic symptoms
- Her husband died 3 years ago

PAST PSYCHIATRIC HISTORY

- Two admissions when she was treated with ECT. Unable to remember dates of admission or number of treatments. Thinks that she has had antidepressant medication of nortryptiline and moclobemide
- Has had ECT two times a week in past – ? when

RELEVANT NEGATIVES

No psychotic symptoms, drug or alcohol abuse.

CONSEQUENCES

Lives alone, finding it an increased effort to go cooking and shopping. Using a cleaner every week.

MANAGEMENT SO FAR

ECT – two treatments a week of unilateral ECT.

FAMILY HISTORY

- Mother and father were in retail industry
- Has two sisters and one brother
- No family history of psychiatric illness

PERSONAL HISTORY

Remembers growing up and enjoying school. Left to enter office work and got married shortly afterwards. Her husband was in business and died 3 years ago of cancer. She felt extremely distressed following the first anniversary of her husband's death. Was working in office until retirement age. Had one son and has a grandchild. The son lives locally and is supportive. She is living off a pension.

PAST MEDICAL HISTORY

- Had an operation on her leg 3 months ago after she fell and it became infected
- No history of hypertension, cardiac or cerebrovascular disease

CIGARETTES

Does not smoke.

FORENSIC

Nil.

PREMORBID PERSONALITY

Usually enjoys company but not when she is feeling depressed

Very clean and particular about household. Had been dependent on her husband who was very supportive of her.

MENTAL STATE EXAMINATION

- Appearance and behaviour – smartly dressed elderly lady with glasses, matching handbag, movements were quite slow, cooperative and pleasant
- Speech was slow and hesitant and she often said 'I don't remember' in response to questions
- Mood 'not very happy'
- Affect – tearful, dysthymic, congruent
- No deliberate self harm, suicidal ideation or intent
- Thought content was mainly preoccupied with self-blaming, guilt, worry about forgetting things, concern that the ECT may not work. No guilt, hypochondriacal or nihilistic delusions
- No obsessive compulsive symptoms
- Perceptions – nil abnormal elicited, not objectively hallucinating
- Cognition – Mini-Mental State testing gave a score of 27/30 with abnormalities in short-term memory testing only. Digit span was five digits forward and four backward, no abnormalities of parietal lobe functioning, no abnormalities of frontal lobe functioning (frontal lobe functioning fist/palm/side, sequencing), verbal fluency (20 animals in 1 min), interpretations of proverbs normal, no apraxia or aphasia
- Insight – wants to get well, believes that her nervous system is at fault and she needs help

ON EXAMINATION

Exclude any endocrine abnormalities, cardiovascular and central nervous system. Leg shows signs of healing ulcer. Some osteoarthritis on hands and feet.

SUMMARY

An 82-year-old widow who was admitted 3 weeks ago following several months of being unable to cope due to depressive symptoms. Has had several admissions to hospital in the past for depression and was treated with ECT. No family history of psychiatric illness. After her husband's death she found the business affairs difficult to manage. Precipitants to her admission include the death of her husband 3 years ago, her recent admission to hospital for the ulcerated leg and family concern for her well-being. Her admission may have caused a loss of confidence in her ability to cope on her own. She may have been unable to meet her exacting standards of household cleanliness and started to feel guilty. She has a supportive family and possible difficulties on discharge from hospital would be going to live on her own again.

DISCUSSION ISSUES

- Diagnosis
- Exclude dementia
- Differentiation of depression from dementia
- Types of depression
- Use of ECT in the elderly, side effects
- Role of maintenance ECT
- Type of antidepressant to use in the elderly

1.3 BIPOLAR AFFECTIVE DISORDER

IDENTIFICATION

Age, sex, marital status, job, involuntary or voluntary admission.

ISSUES

Management of patient who is currently manic, depressed, issues of non-compliance, disruption of adult roles or negotiating developmental requirements of adolescence or young adulthood due to illness, treatment resistance.

DIFFICULTIES

During the interview s/he was disinhibited (as evidenced by ...), irritable (as evidenced by ...), distractible (as evidenced by ...), restless (as evidenced by ...).

REFERRAL

Self, police, relative, Mental Health Act.

HISTORY OF PRESENTING COMPLAINT

Use the mnemonic *GREAT SAD*

Grandiose
Racing thoughts
Euphoria
Activities increased
Talkative
Sleep decreased, Sex increased
Activities self damaging and increased e.g. binge, spend, impulse
Distractible

ONSET

Weeks, decreased sleep, escalates prior to admission.

PRECIPITANTS

Forensic, self-damaging behaviour, life event, poor or non-compliance, drug or alcohol related, seasonal: spring, autumn.

SEVERITY

- Hypomania – change in functioning observed by others but often not self/not psychotic
- Mania – impaired occupational functioning/psychotic

RELEVANT NEGATIVES

Drug and alcohol, deliberate self harm, depression, schizophrenia.

CONSEQUENCES

- Behaviour dangerous, disinhibited, e.g. spend, sex, drug, alcohol
- Social, marital, occupational, forensic and financial

FAMILY HISTORY

- Affective disorder 20–25%
- Genetics – increase of bipolar and unipolar disorders in first-degree relatives
- Male = female bipolar disorder
- Suicide, drug and alcohol

PERSONAL HISTORY

History of axis II and arrested maturation if severe illness.

PAST MEDICAL HISTORY

- Complications of medication, e.g. lithium – check renal, thyroid
- Carbamazepine and valproate – check haematology, liver function
- Secondary mania due to drugs, stimulants, steroids, L-dopa, thyroxine, CNS disease, postencephalitic, tumour, multiple sclerosis, HIV, encephalitis, CVS, CVA

PAST PSYCHIATRIC HISTORY

- Past episodes, seasonal, age of onset, cycles, drugs, depression, delusions, deliberate self harm

- Interepisode functioning
- Past treatment with lithium, carbamazepine, valproate, ECT
- Ask about side effects with treatments, e.g. toxicity
- Which treatments were most successful?
- Present maintenance and compliance

SUBSTANCE ABUSE

High comorbidity, disinhibited, Winokur depressive spectrum, self medication.

FORENSIC AND SOCIAL

Support, expressed emotion, enmeshed, dangerousness.

PREMORBID PERSONALITY

Arrested development, change from premorbid personality, defence style.

CRITERIA FOR MANIC EPISODE   Modified with permission from the Diagnostic and Statistical Manual of Mental Disorders, Fourth Edition. Copyright 1994 American Psychiatric Association.

A. A distinct period of abnormally and persistently elevated, expansive or irritable mood, lasting at least 1 week (or any duration if hospitalization is necessary).

B. During the period of mood disturbance, three (or more) of the following symptoms have persisted (four if the mood is only irritable) and have been present to a significant degree:

- Inflated self esteem or grandiosity
- Decreased need for sleep (e.g. feels rested after only 3 hours of sleep)
- More talkative than usual or pressure to keep talking
- Flight of ideas or subjective experience that thoughts are racing
- Distractibility (i.e. attention too easily drawn to unimportant or irrelevant external stimuli)
- Increase in goal-directed activity (either socially at work or school or sexually) or psychomotor agitation
- Excessive involvement in pleasurable activities that have a high risk for painful consequences (e.g. engaging in unrestrained buying sprees, sexual indiscretions or foolish business investments)

C. The symptoms do not reach criteria for a Mixed Episode

D. The mood disturbance is sufficiently severe to cause marked impairment in occupational functioning or in usual social activities or relationships with others or to necessitate hospitalization to prevent harm to self or others, or there are psychotic features.

E. The symptoms are not due to the direct physiological effects of a substance (e.g. a drug of abuse, a medication or other treatment) or a general medical condition (e.g. hyperthyroidism)

CRITERIA FOR HYPOMANIC EPISODE   Modified with permission from the Diagnostic and Statistical Manual of Mental Disorders, Fourth Edition. Copyright 1994 American Psychiatric Association.

A. A distinct period of persistently elevated, expansive or irritable mood, lasting throughout at least 4 days that is clearly different from the usual non-depressed mood.

B. During the period of mood disturbance three (or more) of the following symptoms have persisted (four if the mood is only irritable) and have been present to a significant degree:

- Inflated self esteem or grandiosity
- Decreased need for sleep (e.g. feels rested after only 3 hours of sleep)
- More talkative than usual or pressure to keep talking
- Flight of ideas or subjective experience that thoughts are racing
- Distractibility (i.e. attention easily drawn to unimportant or irrelevant external stimuli)
- Increase in goal directed activity (either socially, at work or school, or sexually) or psychomotor agitation
- Excessive involvement in pleasurable activities that have a high potential for painful consequences (e.g. person engages in unrestrained buying sprees, sexual indiscretions, or foolish business investments)

C. The episode is associated with an unequivocal change in functioning that is uncharacteristic of the person when not symptomatic.

D. The disturbance in mood and the change in functioning are observable by others.

E. The episode is not severe enough episode to cause marked impairment in social and occupational functioning or to hospitalize and there are no psychotic features.

F. The symptoms are not due to direct physiological effects of a substance (e.g. a drug of abuse, or medication or other treatment) or a general medical condition (e.g. hyperthyroidism).

DIFFERENTIAL DIAGNOSIS OF MANIA

- Mood disorder due to a general medical condition, e.g. HIV, epilepsy, Huntington's, neurosyphilis, multiple sclerosis, Cushing's, SLE, vitamin deficiencies
- Substance-induced mood disorder, amphetamines, baclofen, bromide, bromocriptine, cimetidine, cocaine, CS, disulfiram, hallucinogens, hydralazine, L-dopa, isoniazid, procyclidine, etc
- Hypomanic episodes
- Major depression with irritable mood
- Mixed episodes
- Attention deficit and hyperactivity disorder

For a young patient think of schizophrenia, schizoaffective disorder, drugs, organic, cyclothymia, personality disorder, borderline, narcissitic, brief reactive psychosis, depression.

For an old patient think of dementia, frontal lobe damage, delirium, drug toxicity.

MANAGEMENT ISSUES

Safety and dangerousness

Mental Health Act and setting, limit damage to self, others and reputation.

Clarify diagnosis

- Observations, disability
- Exclude differential diagnosis

SPECIAL INVESTIGATIONS

To exclude ... I would do ...

FBC, ESR, B$_{12}$, folate, UE, LFT, Ca, PO$_4$, TFT, HIV, VDRL, HEPB/C, urinary drug screen, pregnancy test (women), CT, MRI, EEG if indicated.

Lithium work up – TFT, ECG, UE's.

- Collateral history, relations, review medical notes... in order to find out ....
- Role of other professionals – to do what?

Establish a therapeutic alliance

Can be difficult due to mental state however essential to maximize compliance.

Decrease symptoms and treatment using a biopsychosocial model

- Biological – symptom control, (diazepam, haloperidol). May need seclusion, physical constraint. Female contraception and HIV
- Psychosocial – limit setting stimuli, ward milieu, monitor staff reactions

Aim to restore to maximum level of functioning

SHORT-TERM MANAGEMENT

- Safety
- Decrease symptoms using a biopsychosocial approach
- Behaviour, symptoms – neuroleptics and benzodiazepines
- Introduce lithium after work up – if no success then consider carbamazepine or valproate or combination of two mood stabilisers

TREATMENT

- Chlorpromazine 50–100 mg 2–4 hourly or haloperidol 5–10 mg 2 hourly
- Start lithium 750–1000 mg daily and build up to therapeutic level 0.8–1.2 mmol/litre and maintenance level of 0.6–1.0 mmol/litre
- Decrease the antipsychotics as the lithium levels are therapeutic
- Blood lithium – weekly then 12 hours after last dose
- CARE with sodium level, e.g. diuretic, nutrition, exercise, emesis, diarrhoea

Side effects of lithium

- Gastrointestinal – nausea, vomiting, abdominal pain, diarrhoea – slow release, with meals
- Tremor – can treat with 20 mg propanolol
- Polyuria and polydipsia
- Hypothyroid
- Teratogenic effects – cardiovascular system
- Acne, weight gain, anorexia, increased white cell count
- Divide dose if giving > 1g daily to avoid nephrotoxicity
- Decrease antipsychotics once a therapeutic level is reached
- Interactions with lithium include NSAIDs, thiazide diuretics and ACE inhibitors

Psychosocial

- Control milieu, decrease mania and increase insight, supportive education, family support and counselling, build rapport and alliance for post discharge, developmental and psychodynamic issues
- Genograms of family history going back at least two generations – check cousins, aunts, uncles and grandparents

LONG-TERM MANAGEMENT

Pharmacological maintenance

First episode 9 months, more than two episodes – long-term maintenance. After the first manic episode, there is a 50% chance of recurrence without lithium treatment in the first 3 years after the episode.

Lithium

- Monitor UEs, ECG, TFT, lithium levels, side effects
- May need to add in antipsychotic or antidepressant at times
- CARE as antidepressant medication may precipitate mania
- Some patients may need small doses of antipsychotic medication

Carbamazepine if poor response to lithium, mixed episodes or rapid cycling 200 mg bd start and build up to 1200–1600 mg daily
- Side effects – drowsy, ataxia, slurred speech, blurred vision
- Report fever, sore throat ulcers, rash or bruising – e.g. leucopenia or hepatic hypersensitivity occurs in first month of treatment
- Monitor FBC, UE, LFT's

Valproate – if poor response to lithium, carbamazepine, mixed episodes, rapid cycling
- Start 400 mg bd and increase to 1000–2500 mg
- Side effects – gastric irritation

Psychosocial

- Pregnancy risk – care with lithium – likelihood of recurrence, family support.
- Issues, autonomy, stigma, insight, anger, denial, despair.
- Risk of suicide

Multidisciplinary team

Relapse

Maintainance

Use of time lines, e.g. mood, exercise, sleep.

Rehabilitation

Compliance

Optimum level of functioning

Prognosis

1.4 BIPOLAR AFFECTIVE DISORDER CASE

IDENTIFICATION

James is a 30-year-old, single, English man who claims to be a voluntary patient.

ISSUES

- The main issues in the case are management of bipolar affective disorder - currently manic
- The main difficulties during the interview were that the patient was expansive and over inclusive

REFERRAL

The referral was via the police in that James said the police brought him into hospital as he was screaming at the public.

HISTORY OF PRESENTING COMPLAINT

- 'Saw ship on horizon from the United States President which was coming to pick me up and take me to the States'
- Believes that he is the Messiah and has the power to heal people
- Describes racing thoughts 'supersonic'
- Has had an increase in debt over the last year but has not recently spent more money
- Is talkative and distractible
- Sleep pattern decreased, energy increased, libido increased

PAST PSYCHIATRIC HISTORY

- Has a history of depression 3 years ago when he was treated with lithium and fluoxetine. At the time described feeling down, low mood, appetite poor, interrupted sleep, decreased energy, occasional suicidal ideation, no guilt, loss of interest in things
- There is no history of deliberate self harm
- He continued to take lithium until 2 years ago when he stopped as he no longer felt depressed

RELEVANT NEGATIVES

First rank symptoms, drinks alcohol occasionally, has abused cannabis in the past.

CONSEQUENCES

As a consequence of his admission he has had contact with his family.

CURRENT TREATMENT

Haloperidol.

FAMILY HISTORY

His father suffered from bipolar affective disorder.

PERSONAL HISTORY

- He had an unremarkable upbringing, apart from a period in America, due to his father's job when he was in his teens
- He has had many friends although no serious relationships. He is currently on sickness benefit
- There is no past medical history of note
- He smokes cigarettes and has had several altercations with the police

PREMORBID PERSONALITY

He finds he is often restless; Enjoys painting and sculpture.

MENTAL STATE EXAMINATION

- Thin young man, casually dressed, smoking a cigarette and drinking coffee
- His speech was expansive and rapid and was difficult to interrupt at times. There was no flight of ideas, punning or clanging
- His mood he described as 'fantastic' and his affect was expansive and irritable at times
- There was no suicidal ideation or intent
- Thought content was grandiose - felt he was the Messiah and a talented actor
- No disorder of thought possession
- Perceptions - not objectively hallucinating and nil abnormal elicited
- Cognition - 26/30 in the mini Mental State Exam. Abnormalities in short-term memory testing and the date being incorrect

- No other abnormalities of parietal, frontal lobes
- Insight - he feels he is cured and has no need to be in hospital although he states he will continue to see a psychiatrist after discharge

ON EXAMINATION

There were no signs of endocrine abnormalities, no extrapyramidal side effects, lying and standing blood pressure were within normal limits, no sign of alcohol or drug abuse.

SUMMARY

A 30-year-old admitted after a behavioural disturbance with symptoms of mania (grandiose delusions, rapid thought, decreased sleep, increase in activities, increase energy and libido). He has a past psychiatric history of depression when he was treated with lithium and an antipsychotic. No recent drug or alcohol abuse. There is a family history of bipolar affective disorder.

Possible precipitants include not having been on any medication for 2 years. He is currently unable to care for himself as his judgement is impaired. He currently agrees that he needs medication although does not feel unwell. Compliance would be a major issue in his continuing care. His illness is impacting on his ability to have meaningful relationships with other people which is important as part of his life stage.

DISCUSSION ISSUES

- Safety
- Compliance and non-compliance with medication
- Role of lithium, valproate, carbamazepine and side effects
- Role of community and key workers
- Prognosis
- Management of treatment resistant mania

MANAGEMENT OF TREATMENT RESISTANT MANIA

- Use of medication
- Biopsychosocial approach
- Look for contributing:
    Patient factors
    Drug factors
    Social factors

1.5 POST PARTUM PROBLEMS

IDENTIFICATION

Post partum psychosis, primiparous versus multiparous, marital status, occupation.

ISSUES

Safety, management of child and marital issues.

DIFFICULTIES

Mother/child interaction.

REFERRAL

Self, spouse, midwife, obstetrician, GP, early childhood nurse, paediatrician, emergency department, liaison.

HISTORY OF PRESENTING COMPLAINT

- Presenting symptoms
- Prodromal features – insomnia, restlessness, fatigue, lability, tearfulness
- Psychotic – affective – 80% focus on babies health and welfare, schizophrenia first episode and relapse
- Suicidality, infanticidality
- Depression – 10–15% of women have endogenous features
- Post partum blues – 3–4 days tearful, labile
- Depressed withdrawal, sleep disturbance, irritability, preoccupied, overwhelmed with the baby
- Onset and course
- Treatment to date and response

MOTHER

- History of pregnancy, primiparous, multiparous, planned, unplanned, personal expectations, cultural expectation, medical complications, e.g. eclampsia, thyroid, cardiovascular, renal, hepatic
- Drug and alcohol – depression, abuse, withdrawal, self medication, dysphoria, risk HIV and hepatitis

BABY

Birth weight, temperament of baby, feed, sleep, response, crying.

RELEVANT NEGATIVES

Infanticidality, drugs and alcohol, psychotic symptoms, obsessive compulsive disorder.

CONSEQUENCES

MOTHER

- Dangerousness, deliberate self harm
- Severity – psychosis, impaired reality testing

BABY

Neglect of child, breast feeding.

FAMILY

Effect on family of new child, ill parent, etc.

FAMILY HISTORY

Depression, anxiety, psychosis, drug and alcohol, suicide and deliberate self harm.

PERSONAL HISTORY

- Early development, parenting experience, abuse, separation, rejection, loss, dysfunction, school, work, relationships, marital, *de facto* relationship, current relationship with family
- Social supports – family, marital, friends, housing finance, network, social class, life events, lack rites of transition

PREMORBID PERSONALITY

Habitual defences, ego strength, affect, impulsivity, identity, self efficacy, self harm.

MENTAL STATE EXAMINATION

- Typical of puerperal psychosis is perplexity, sudden onset, fluctuation between depression and mania, disorganized, confused, disorientated
- Mood – depressed, elevated, fluctuating, inappropriate labile affect
- Cognitions – hopeless, helpless, anhedonia, decreased worth and self esteem, guilt, negative view of self, world and future, suicide and infanticide, preoccupied with baby being deceased, deformed and diseased; overvalued ideas, delusions and delirium
- Perceptions, cognition and insight

ON EXAMINATION

Exclude hypothyroid, anaemia, endocrine, cardiovascular and central nervous system abnormalities.

DIFFERENTIAL DIAGNOSIS

- Post partum psychosis – psychotic depression, mania, schizophrenia, organic
- Depression
- Delirium
- Adjustment reaction
- Generalized anxiety disorder, obsessive compulsive disorder
- Eclampsia – with convulsions, hypothyroidism, substance abuse withdrawal, Cushing's

---

MANAGEMENT

Safety and dangerousness

Mental Health Act and setting, mother and child, inpatient.

- Safety of mother and child, physical, neglect, self care, nutrition and psychological
- Aim to decrease symptoms, support mother and child, bond
- Inpatient – suicidal, infanticidal, medical, admit to mother and baby unit
- Outpatient – good social supports, supervision, no safety issues, therapeutic alliance

SPECIAL INVESTIGATIONS

To exclude ... I would do ...

Physical examination – blood pressure, pulse, temperature, respiratory rate.

Special Investigations: FBC, ESR, UE's, B_{12}, folate, LFT, Ca, Mg, TFT, glucose, drug screen, ECG, CXR, EEG, CT.

Clarify primary diagnosis

Corroborative history, spouse, partner, friends, old notes.

- Observations and disability, regular review of mental state
- Exclude differential diagnosis
- Collateral history and additional sources of information to find out what ...? Interview with husband/spouse/partner
- Role of other professionals – to do what?

Establish a therapeutic alliance

Treat with a biopsychosocial model

- Biological – assessment of depression, treat with appropriate antidepressant, ECT, mood stabilizer, neuroleptics
- Psychosis – neuroleptic and mood stabilizers
- Contraception
- Psychological – psychosocial assessment of psychiatric and obstetric history
- Educative and parent skills, support and practical, marital and CBT
- Social – support increased, acknowledge stress, improve network for carer, child care, self help, advocacy

Restore to optimum level of functioning

LONG-TERM MANAGEMENT

- Safety
- Goals to maintain, prevent relapse, rehabilitation, parenting skills

Treatment

- Biological – depending on breast feeding, antidepressants, e.g. dothiepin (normal dose range), fluoxetine, neuroleptics – if necessary
- Contraception
- Breast feed – care with sedation, lithium toxicity, lethargy and weight loss
- Psychological – supportive, dynamic, inpatient, conflicts in self esteem and relationships, therapeutic alliance
- Care of infant: ensure adequate mother – infant attachment

- Social – network support and self help, monitor at risk children and advocacy
- Prognosis – bipolar affective disorder, 50% recurrence in future pregnancies
- Difficulties – family, legal, forensic, support, developmental stage, drugs and alcohol, parenting and monitor compliance

AETIOLOGY

- Infection, drugs, toxaemia and blood loss.

PREGNANCY

- Minor psychological symptoms – 66% of women have anxiety in first and last trimesters
- 10% depressed during pregnancy – associated with past history of depression, previous abortion, pregnancy unwanted, marital conflict and anxieties about the foetus – fatigue, irritability, increased neuroticism scores
- Depression in the last trimester may persist as postnatal depression

MANAGEMENT

Increased support by services and family, drug treatment avoided in first trimester, marital therapy.

PUERPERAL PSYCHOSIS

- 1.5 per 1000 deliveries, primiparous, past history of manic depression – 20–40 % chance of puerperal psychosis, first child, Caesarean, psychosocial factors
- Genetic factors – family history of major psychiatric disorder predisposes to puerperal psychosis
- Biochemistry – decrease of progesterone and oestrogen on tryptophan metabolism
- Psychodynamic factors – own parenting, etc
- Clinical features – affective psychoses 70% and schizophrenia 25%, organic rare
- Affective psychosis mainly depressive
- Unlikely to be a separate entity as family history of psychotic disorder is as common in non-puerperal psychosis, increased incidence of psychosis before and after the pregnancy and puerperal period also, manic depressive have ten times risk of developing a puerperal psychosis compared with a normal population. Clinical syndromes resemble the psychoses occurring at other times
- Distinct clinical picture of puerperal psychosis – prodromal period 2 days post partum with insomnia, irritability, restlessness, refusal of food and depression
- Acute onset of confusion, excitability, over activity, hallucinations, fatiguability, labile mood, preoccupations, delusions concerning the baby. Elation and grandiosity and

schizophrenic symptoms are common, delusions occur in 50% of patients and hallucinations in about 25%
- Onset within 2 weeks of birth

Prognosis

- 70% recover fully, affective have a better prognosis
- Future risk of psychosis in puerperal periods is risk of psychosis at any future time is 50%
- Poor prognosis – positive family history, schizophrenia, neurotic personality, marital problems
- Good prognosis – good premorbid adjustment and supportive family

PUERPERAL DEPRESSION

- 10–15% of women in first month – associated with increased age, difficulties with role model attachments, problems in relationships with mother and father in law and marital conflict, mixed feelings about the baby, physical problems in pregnancy and perinatal period and a tendency to be more neurotic personalities
- Life event – changes in financial, social and marital status, lack of support from family
- Kumar and Robson (1984) – incidence of depression, psychosocial factors. Antenatal – marital problems, ambivalence, TOP, bereavement; Postnatal – marital problems, ambivalence, problems with mother, psychiatric problem with spouse, premature baby
- Typically tearful and irritable, associated symptoms may include feeling tired, despondent and anxious with worry about ability to cope with baby, fear for own and babies health, economic stressors imposed by child
- 50% are depressed 6 months after onset

POST PARTUM BLUES

- 50% of women on third day last for up to 10 days, primiparous and premenstrual tension associated factors – similar to women after major and minor surgery
- Clinical features – weeping, depressed and irritable, and feeling separate and distant from the baby, insomnia, poor concentration. Weight loss, decreased thirst and increased sodium retention

MANAGEMENT

- Psychosis – admit due to danger to baby – together and build up a relationship
- Drugs – for symptoms – care with breast feeding
- Psychotherapy – supportive and marital
- Depression – antidepressant

- TOP – 0.3% per 1000 terminations – psychiatric illness (one-fifth of puerperal psychosis rate). If increased risk for psychiatric indications for termination then increased risk of post-termination depression – 7%
- If the termination is advised and performed for depression 70% improve in mood, 23% remain depressed, 7% worse
- Married women refused a termination regret continuing the pregnancy more than having a termination

DRUGS DURING PREGNANCY AND LACTATION

PREGNANCY

- Risks in pregnancy – first trimester – gross anatomical damage is most likely to occur in the first trimester during the period of organogenesis
- Second trimester – central nervous system development of foetus
- Third trimester – high risk of loading foetus with drugs prelabour with withdrawal at birth
- Start with non-pharmacological support, e.g. psychotherapy, environmental manipulation, family therapy, cognitive behavioural therapy
- Minimum effective dose
- Antidepressants – low dose and increase slowly

IN PREGNANCY, WHEN CHOOSING ANTIDEPRESSANTS CONSIDER:

• Teratogenesis	Use TCA / SSRI*
• Withdrawal / toxicity	Isolated case reports
• Obstetric complications/prematurity	Use TCA / Fluoxetine*
• Long-term neurobehavioural sequalae	Use TCA / Fluoxetine*

* on basis of controlled prospective studies

- Tricyclics – previous reports showed limb reduction at birth but prospective studies show no evidence of teratogenesis
- MAOI – possible increased risk of foetal malformation
- SSRIs – no evidence of abnormalities
  Lithium – first trimester causes foetal defects especially of the cardiovascular system
- Valproate and carbamazepine – cause spina bifida, therefore avoid
- Long-acting benzodiazepines – teratogenicity. They cross the placenta and are associated with the floppy infant syndrome characterised by hypotonia, lethargy, sucking difficulties and neonatal withdrawal syndrome, intrauterine growth retardation, tremors, hypertonicity and diarrhoea and vomiting
- Antianxiety drugs and sedatives – avoid long half-life in pregnancy, those with short half life, e.g. temazepam, may be used. May use sedative TCA
- Antipsychotic drugs – if required, use high potency drugs in the first trimester
- Chlorpromazine – crosses the placenta and there is some concern about teratogenic effects
- Barbiturates – increased risk of neonatal withdrawal syndrome.

LACTATION

- Breast feeding – tricyclic antidepressants "safe", but avoid doxepin (long half-life) which may lead to toxicity. Two controlled studies with follow-up (3 years prothiaden, 1 year sertraline)
- Lithium may cause side effects in the infant so monitor for restlessness, weakness and maternal lithium levels – best avoid and use anticonvulsant
- Antipsychotic – galactorrhoea in mother and drowsiness and lethargy in infants
- Phenothiazines can cause flaccidity or drowsiness in infant
- Diazepam – monitor infant for drowsiness as this has long half-life. Use short acting benzodiazepines

1.6 POST PARTUM PROBLEMS CASE

IDENTIFICATION

30-year-old woman, married with two children, housewife, discharged yesterday.

ISSUES

Management of post partum affective disorder.

DIFFICULTIES

Some difficulty in remembering precipitants.

REFERRAL

Referred to hospital during last week of pregnancy when her blood pressure had increased.

HISTORY OF PRESENTING COMPLAINT

- Put onto bedrest and had baby via a normal vaginal delivery. Required stitches, birth took 4 hours
- On the third day felt weepy and tearful. Remembers hearing voices but is unsure of their content. Did not recognize the three voices. Thought she may have seen three people approach her but was unsure whether this was real. Was concerned that the baby may be harmed and threatened and was preoccupied with protecting the baby
- At this time her appetite was poor and she was not sleeping, interest was good, no guilty feelings, concentration poor, energy levels normal, restless, no suicidal ideation or intent. No risk to the baby. The baby was a planned one and the marital relationship is good

PAST PSYCHIATRIC HISTORY

- Four years ago had first child which was planned, good marital relationship
- After an 18 hour labour and forceps delivery she felt full of energy and experienced the Lord talking to her. The television was giving her messages. She was talking fast, had the

experience of her thoughts racing and was restless and distractible. She was started on thioridazine and discharged. About 1 week later she was feeling low and suicidal, took an overdose of the medication. She was admitted to a psychiatric hospital and treated with antidepressant medication and then ECT - eight sessions when that did not work

- After discharge saw a psychiatrist every 3 months and has been on no medication in the last 2 years

RELEVANT NEGATIVES

Not at risk to herself or baby. No evidence of alcohol, drug abuse or schizophrenia.

CONSEQUENCES

She has now returned home and her husband has some time off work to help. A relative is also staying with them. She is breast feeding the baby. She is also receiving help with her other child.

MANAGEMENT SO FAR

Has been on thioridazine.

FAMILY HISTORY

One aunt had history of affective disorder and was depressed.

PERSONAL HISTORY

Was looked after by grandparents from age of 5 years as her parents were divorced. Went to live with father when he remarried. Relationship with father is supportive and she describes him as caring. No relationship with her mother since age of 11 years. On leaving school met husband at first job as a receptionist. Married and had first child. Had a miscarriage 3 years afterwards. Describes her relationship as supportive. Husband works in Information Technology. Financially no problems.

PAST MEDICAL HISTORY

Nil of note.

CIGARETTES/ALCOHOL

Nil.

FORENSIC HISTORY

Nil.

PREMORBID PERSONALITY

Describes herself as quiet, friendly and independent. Able to do things for herself and is busy. Copes by writing things down if she is unsure of what to do. Has a few close friends and confides in her husband mainly.

MENTAL STATE EXAMINATION

- Appearance and behaviour - casually dressed, hair up, make up and jewellery
- No abnormal mannerisms or movements
- Speech coherent, spontaneous, no formal thought disorder
- Mood described as 'good'
- Affect was euthymic and mood congruent with good range and reactivity
- No suicidal ideation or intent
- Thought content mainly preoccupied with breast feeding her son
- No delusions
- No disorder of thought possession
- No abnormal perceptions elicited or objectively hallucinating
- Cognition grossly intact
- Insight concerned with getting better. Feels she was treated promptly and so was not as ill as last time. Agrees to decrease medication slowly and continue to see a psychiatrist. Had been warned about possibility of becoming ill again with another pregnancy

ON EXAMINATION

Blood pressure 120/60, no signs of infection, or endocrine abnormalities.

SUMMARY

A 30-year-old, married woman with two children who was recently discharged from a brief admission after the birth of her second child when she experienced some psychotic symptoms and mood disturbance. There is a past psychiatric history of affective disorder after the birth of her first child which resulted in a long admission and treatment with ECT.

There is a family history of affective disorder. The pregnancy was complicated by eclampsia prior to birth and separation from the family as a result of this. The birth of her second child may have reminded her of the severity of the illness after her first child. She has good family support and feels bonded to her newborn baby. She has a mature coping style and uses humour; anticipates problems and how to deal with them. She appears realistic about difficulties facing her.

DISCUSSION

- Diagnosis
- Differential diagnosis
- Safety of mother and baby – assessment of
- Therapeutic alliance
- Use of medication in pregnancy and when breast feeding
- Use of ECT
- Risk of recurrence of illness with and without subsequent pregnancies
- Assessment of bonding of mother and child

PSYCHOSIS

2.1 FIRST ADMISSION PSYCHOSIS

IDENTIFICATION

Age, sex, marital status, occupation, culture.

REFERRED

Rarely self, police, family, Mental Health Act.

ISSUES

Onset of psychotic illness, impact on developmental stage, diagnostic ambiguity, substance abuse, suicide, management of dangerousness, risk of violence, insight, prevention of secondary morbidity. Psychoeducation, early development of therapeutic alliance and engagement. Impact on the family.

DIFFICULTIES

Safety, veracity, lack of insight, difficulties in engagement.

HISTORY OF PRESENTING COMPLAINT

- Onset – why now?
- Course, duration, precipitants
- What is the relationship of symptoms to any recent major stressors?

Use mnemonics

(See overleaf)

DEPRESSION

Use mnemonic *SIGE CAPS*

Sleep disturbed
Interest diminished
Guilt
Energy decreased
Concentration decreased
Appetite and weight up or down
Psychomotor retardation or agitation
Suicide

SCHIZOPHRENIA

Use mnemonic *ACID PH SODAS*

Affect
Catatonic
Incoherent language or speech
Delusions
Prominent **H**allucinations
Rule out **S**chizoaffective
Rule out **O**rganic
Decline in functioning
Autism – consider
Six months

MANIA

Use mnemonic *GREAT SAD*

Grandiose
Racing thoughts
Euphoria
Activities increased
Talkative
Sleep decreased, Sex increased
Activities are self damaging and increased e.g., binge, spend, impulse
Distractible

RELEVANT NEGATIVES

Drugs and alcohol, head injury, epilepsy, deliberate self harm.

CURRENT TREATMENT

Treatment so far and patient's attitude/compliance to medication.

CONSEQUENCES

Consequences of symptoms on self, family, finances, accommodation, relationships, occupational functioning. Effect of substance abuse.

FAMILY HISTORY

Psychosis, affective disorder, suicide. Assessment of support within family.

PERSONAL HISTORY

- Pregnancy, birth, developmental milestones, school, interpersonal and psychosexual development
- Any evidence of decline in social, occupational, interpersonal and behaviour?
- Failure to reach expected levels of achievement

PAST MEDICAL HISTORY

Perinatal trauma, head injury, epilepsy, medication and iatrogenic.

PAST PSYCHIATRIC HISTORY

- Prodromal behaviour, past psychiatric disorder, deliberate self harm
- Previous psychiatric assessments
- Childhood learning difficulties

FORENSIC

May be first indication that there is something wrong if get into trouble about behaviour which is unusual or bizarre.

PREMORBID PERSONALITY

- Establish previous level of functioning
- Schizoid, schizotypal

MENTAL STATE EXAMINATION

- Appearance, incoherence, mood, affect, psychotic features, insight, cognition, movement disorders, tardive dyskinesia
- Exclude drug and alcohol intoxication

ON EXAMINATION

- Stigmata of drug and alcohol abuse, tattoos, needles
- Central nervous system signs, pulse, blood pressure, temperature

DIFFERENTIAL DIAGNOSIS Modified with permission from the Diagnostic and Statistical Manual of Mental Disorders, Fourth Edition. Copyright 1994 American Psychiatric Association.

- Psychotic disorder due to a general medical condition*
- Delirium
- Dementia
- Substance-induced psychotic disorder, e.g. amphetamines, cocaine, PCP; intoxication with substances e.g. alcohol, cannabis, opioids, sedatives, hypnotics, anxiolytics; withdrawal from substances e.g. alcohol, sedatives, hypnotics and anxiolytics.
- Substance-induced delirium
- Substance-induced dementia
- Mood disorder with psychotic features
- Schizoaffective disorder
- Schizophreniform disorder
- Brief reactive psychosis
- Delusional disorder
- Psychotic disorder not otherwise specified
- Pervasive developmental disorders
- Schizoid, schizotypal, paranoid personality disorder
- Medication induced, e.g. L-dopa or beta blockers
- Post partum psychosis

*Psychotic disorder due to general medical condition

- Neurological, e.g. neoplasms, cerebrovascular disease, Huntington's disease, epilepsy, auditory nerve injury, deafness, migraine, CNS infections, Alzheimer's, multiple sclerosis, multi-infarct dementia
- Endocrine, e.g. hyper- and hypothyroidism, hyper- and hypoparathyroidism, hypoadrenocorticism
- Metabolic, e.g. hypoxia, hypercarbia, hypoglycaemia, fluid or electrolyte imbalances, hepatic or renal disease
- Autoimmune, e.g. systemic lupus erythematosus

MANAGEMENT

Safety and dangerousness

- Mental Health Act and setting/community
- Admit if dangerous, serious disorganization, fearful affect, agitation, presumed organic aetiology, concurrent substance abuse and depleted family resources

Clarify diagnosis (may be difficult)

Symptom clarity and stability are poor with up to 50% of patients changing operational diagnosis from episode one to two. Many early intervention centres use 'psychosis' as a low stigma and acceptable diagnosis in the first episode. Treat comorbidity, e.g. depression, anxiety, post-traumatic stress disorder, drug and alcohol abuse.

- Observations behaviour, disability, level of functioning. Regular review of mental state
- Exclude differential diagnosis

SPECIAL INVESTIGATIONS

To exclude ... I would do ...

FBC, UE, CR, LFT, TFT, glucose, Ca, PO_4, HIV, VDRL, B_{12}, folate, ESR, hepatitis, urinary drug screen, EEG, CT, CXR.

To exclude:

- Substance abuse – urine/drug screen
- Liver function abnormalites – LFTs
- Systemic infection – FBC, ESR, CXR , MSU
- Nutritional – FBC, B_{12}, folate, iron
- CNS abnormalities – MRI, CT
- Encephalitis – LP
- Metabolic disorder – UE's, Creatinine, TFTs
- Cardiac abnormalities – ECG

- Collaborative history and additional sources of information to find out ....
- Role of other professionals – to do what?

Establish a therapeutic alliance

One of the best predictors of outcome in schizophrenia is the development of a stable therapeutic alliance. Specific strategies include:

- Working with patient to explore and test the validity of their beliefs, interpretations and expectations
- A respectful, non-confrontational approach to psychotic material
- Addressing dilemmas involving safety and differences of interpretation between client and treating team
- Working collaboratively with the client to solve their identified problems
- Focus on medium-term not just short-term goals
- Collaborative approach to medication if possible
- Respect for the persons overall quality of life and ambitions

Decrease symptoms using a biopsychosocial model

Biological

- Drug-free period for observation if possible to observe psychopathology

- Initiate treatment, oral/parenteral sedation, seclusion or restraint, nursing
- Symptoms – decrease, effect of ward milieu. Important to separate from chronic patients
- Zuclopenthixol acetate – useful for short-term management of acute psychosis
- Choice of neuroleptic – depends on side effects which can be tolerated for that particular person
- Start low dose neuroleptic and increase slowly, minimize side effects
- May use low dose haloperidol or risperidone
- Olanzapine, clozapine, sertindole
- To avoid side effects use anticholinergics
- Benzodiazepines – useful for sedation
- Lithium – if affective features present or if several neuroleptics unsuccessful
- Antidepressants if depression precedes psychosis but if it is concurrent then antipsychotics alone
- Monitor compliance and side effects
- Information re side effects and education re medication will increase compliance and diminish fear and stigma

Psychological

- Rapport, engagement, therapeutic alliance, empathy, non-judgemental, reassurance and support, attention and unconditional positive regard, supportive therapy
- Meaning of episode
- Explore fears
- Education – early warning signs
- Provide rationale for medication, explain effects and side effects
- Reduce duration of untreated psychosis by increasing access, e.g. promotional outreach services to doctors, schools and counsellors
- Assessment – re long-term needs (personality difficulties, life issues)
- Intervention for comorbid problems

Family therapy

- Beneficial in preventing relapse in the first 9 months after discharge
- Family support and education
- Decrease expressed emotion
- Form a positive working relationship
- Provide structure and stability
- Respect for interpersonal boundaries
- Cognitive restructuring
- Behavioural tasks
- Facilitation of communication
- Focus on the here and now
- Often address guilt, loss, coping with crises and negative symptoms
- Crisis intervention support

Social

Advocacy, assistance, finance, welfare, housing, support, education, self help.

Restore to optimum level of functioning

First episode psychosis patients have a good short-term recovery which gives an opportunity for preventative interventions before the onset of intractable symptoms.

LONG-TERM MANAGEMENT

- Safety
- Multimodal multidisciplinary team

Biological

- Maintenance of medication, e.g. neuroleptic for 2 years for first episode schizophrenia
- Issues for patient in terms of long term compliance with medication

Psychological

- 1–2 years assertive follow up, case manager for care and support
- Establish hope, promote recovery
- Empowerment of patient as expert in their illness experience

Cognitive behavioural therapy

- Monitor symptoms and compliance
- Education and early warning signs, drugs and alcohol

Social

Education, advocacy, self help, social skills, living skills, social supports.

DISCUSSION ISSUES

- Diagnostic criteria
- Precipitants
- Vulnerability, stress vulnerability diathesis
- Treatment – symptoms based approach
- Prognosis
    - 10–15% of people with non-affective psychosis commit suicide
    - Two-thirds of suicides occur in the first 5 years predicted by an awareness of the deteriorative effects of illness in the context of good premorbid adjustment, fear of mental deterioration and hopelessness
    - Chronic depression in 30% of patients with schizophrenia
    - Of those with first episode psychosis, 25% do not have another episode
    - Increasing evidence that each relapse is associated with further functional decline

2.2 SCHIZOPHRENIA

IDENTIFICATION

- Age, sex, marital status, job, involuntary or voluntary status, culture
- Men – early 20s, women late 20s and early 30s

ISSUES

Management of patient, safety and dangerousness, non-compliance, family involvement, rehabilitation, comorbid drug and alcohol use, insight.

DIFFICULTIES

During the interview there were difficulties with communication (as evidenced by ...), veracity.

REFERRAL

Self, outpatients, relative, community, police, forensic.

HISTORY OF PRESENTING COMPLAINT

ONSET

Prodromal? An exacerbation?

PRECIPITANTS

Why now? What has been the change in functioning? What stressors/precipitants?

Use mnemonic *ACID PH SODAS*

*A*ffect
*C*atatonia
*I*ncoherent language or speech
*D*elusions
*P*rominent *H*allucinations
rule out *S*chizoaffective

rule out **O**rganic
Decline in functioning
Autism – consider
Six months

Ask about negative symptoms

PAST PSYCHIATRIC HISTORY

Duration of illness, age of onset, type and effects of treatment so far – compliance, medication and response. Any deliberate self harm?

RELEVANT NEGATIVES

Affective disorder, mood, anxiety, drugs or alcohol, deliberate self harm, suicide, homicide.

CONSEQUENCES

- Suicide, deliberate self harm, aggression
- Family, work, social relationships
- Forensic issues, disabilities, handicap

FAMILY HISTORY

- Genetic component
- Relationship to the person with schizophrenia – parent 5%, sibling 10%, child of one person with schizophrenia 14%, child of two people with schizophrenia 46%
- Inheritance – not a specific mode, some vulnerability and environmental factors lead to expression as schizophrenia

PERSONAL HISTORY

Decline in functioning, mental retardation, learning difficulties, epilepsy.

PAST MEDICAL HISTORY

- Perinatal trauma, head injury, epilepsy
- Concurrent medical conditions – aetiology, effect, treatment response and prognosis
- Consequences of drug and alcohol – hepatitis, overdose, HIV, forensic

SOCIAL SUPPORTS

Family, agency, friends, self help.

PREMORBID PERSONALITY

Schizoid, schizotypal.

MENTAL STATE EXAMINATION

Appearance affect, movement disorders, e.g. tardive dyskinesia, catatonia, incoherence, formal thought disorder, psychosis, cognition, insight.

ON PHYSICAL EXAMINATION

Signs of drugs and alcohol abuse, tattoos, needles. Central nervous systems signs, movement disorders, pulse, blood pressure

DIAGNOSTIC CRITERIA FOR SCHIZOPHRENIA Modified with permission from the Diagnostic and Statistical Manual of Mental Disorders, Fourth Edition. Copyright 1994 American Psychiatric Association.

A. Characteristic symptoms: two (or more) of the following, each present for a significant portion of time during a 1 month period (or less if successfully treated):

- Delusions
- Hallucinations
- Disorganized speech, e.g. frequent derailment or incoherence
- Grossly disorganized or catatonic behaviour
- Negative symptoms, i.e. affective flattening, alogia, avolition

Note: only one criterion A symptom is required if delusions are bizarre or hallucinations consist of a voice keeping up a running commentary on the persons behaviour or thoughts or two or more voices conversing with each other.

B. Social/occupational dysfunction: For a significant portion of the time since the onset of the disturbance, one or more major areas of functioning such as work, interpersonal relationships, or self care are markedly below the level achieved prior to the onset (or when the onset is in childhood or adolescence, failure to achieve expected level of interpersonal, academic, or occupational achievement).

C. Duration: continuous signs of the disturbance persist for at least 6 months. This 6-month period must include at least 1 month of symptoms (or less if successfully treated) that meet criterion A (i.e. active phase symptoms) and may include periods of prodromal or residual symptoms. During these prodromal or residual periods, the signs of the disturbance may be manifested by only negative symptoms or two or more symptoms listed in criterion A present in attenuated form (e.g. odd beliefs, unusual perceptual experiences).

D. Schizoaffective and mood disorder exclusion: schizoaffective disorder and mood disorder with psychotic features have been ruled out because either (1) no major depressive, manic or mixed episodes have occurred concurrently with the active-phase symptoms or (2). if mood episodes have occurred during active-phase symptoms their total duration has been brief relative to the duration of the active and residual periods.

E. Substance abuse and general medical condition exclusion: The disturbance is not due to the direct physiological effects of a substance (e.g. drug of abuse, medication) or a general medical condition.

F. Relationship to a pervasive developmental disorder: If there is a history of autistic disorder or another pervasive developmental disorder the additional diagnosis of schizophrenia is made only if prominent delusions or hallucinations are also present for at least a month (or less if successfully treated).

Classification of longitudinal course (can be applied only after at least 1 year has elapsed since the initial onset of active phase symptoms):

Episodic with Interepisode Residual Symptoms (episodes are defined by the reemergence of prominent psychotic symptoms); *also specify if:*

— With Prominent Negative Symptoms

— Episodic with No Interepisode Residual Symptoms

Continuous (prominent psychotic symptoms are present throughout the period of observation); *also specify if:*

— With Prominent Negative Symptoms

— Single Episode in Full Remission

— Other or Unspecified Pattern

PARANOID TYPE   Modified with permission from the Diagnostic and Statistical Manual of Mental Disorders, Fourth Edition. Copyright 1994 American Psychiatric Association.

A type of schizophrenia in which the following criteria are met:

• Preoccupation with one or more delusions or frequent auditory hallucinations
• None of the following are prominent: disorganised speech, disorganized or catatonic behaviour, flat or inappropriate affect

DISORGANISED TYPE   Modified with permission from the Diagnostic and Statistical Manual of Mental Disorders, Fourth Edition. Copyright 1994 American Psychiatric Association.

A type of Schizophrenia in which the following criteria are met:

• All the following are prominent:
  Disorganized speech
  Disorganized behaviour
  Flat or inappropriate affect
• The criteria are not met for catatonic type

CATATONIC TYPE
Modified with permission from the Diagnostic and Statistical Manual of Mental Disorders, Fourth Edition. Copyright 1994 American Psychiatric Association.

A type of schizophrenia in which the clinical picture is dominated by at least two of the following:

- Motoric immobility as evidenced by catalepsy (including waxy flexibility) or stupor
- Excessive motor activity (that is apparently purposeless and not influenced by external stimuli)
- Extreme negativism (an apparently motiveless resistance to all instructions or maintenance of a rigid posture against attempts to be moved) or mutism
- Peculiarities of voluntary movement as evidenced by posturing (voluntary assumption of inappropriate or bizarre postures) stereotyped movements, prominent mannerisms or prominent grimacing
- Echolalia or echopraxia

RESIDUAL TYPE
Modified with permission from the Diagnostic and Statistical Manual of Mental Disorders, Fourth Edition. Copyright 1994 American Psychiatric Association.

A type of schizophrenia in which the following criteria are met:

- Absence of prominent delusions or hallucinations, disorganized speech and grossly disorganized or catatonic behaviour
- There is continuing evidence of disturbance, as indicated by the presence of negative symptoms or two or more symptoms listed in criterion A for Schizophrenia, present in an attenuated form (e.g. odd beliefs, unusual perceptual experiences)

UNDIFFERENTIATED TYPE
Modified with permission from the Diagnostic and Statistical Manual of Mental Disorders, Fourth Edition. Copyright 1994 American Psychiatric Association.

A type of schizophrenia in which symptoms that meet criterion A are present but the criteria are not met for the paranoid, disorganized or catatonic type.

DIFFERENTIAL DIAGNOSIS

- Psychotic disorder due to a general medical condition*
- Delirium
- Dementia
- Substance-induced psychotic disorder, e.g. amphetamines, cocaine, PCP, cannabis, alcohol
- Substance-induced delirium
- Substance-induced dementia
- Mood disorder with psychotic features
- Schizoaffective disorder
- Schizophreniform disorder
- Brief reactive psychosis
- Delusional disorder

- Psychotic disorder not otherwise specified
- Pervasive developmental disorders
- Schizoid, schizotypal, paranoid personality disorder
- Medication induced, e.g. L-dopa or beta blockers

*Psychotic disorder due to general medical condition

- Neurological, e.g. neoplasms, cerebrovascular disease, Huntington's disease, epilepsy, auditory nerve injury, deafness, migraine, CNS infections, Alzheimer's, multiple sclerosis, multi-infarct dementia
- Endocrine, e.g. hyper- and hypothyroidism, hyper- and hypoparathyroidism, hypoadrenocorticism
- Metabolic, e.g. hypoxia, hypercarbia, hypoglycaemia, fluid or electrolyte imbalances, hepatic or renal disease
- Autoimmune, e.g. systemic lupus erythematosus

MANAGEMENT ISSUES

Safety and dangerousness

- Mental Health Act and setting
- Safeguard patient and community and persons reputation
- Provide a structure which reduces stimulation, anxiety and perplexity, removes stress
- Instructions to nursing staff and safety observations
- Care for patient in the least restrictive setting that is safe and allows for effective treatment

Clarify diagnosis

- Observations and disability – collaborative history, old notes, e.g. inpatient/community, observations on ward
- Often comorbid diagnosis of substance abuse or dependence up to 40%.
- Exclude differential diagnosis

SPECIAL INVESTIGATIONS

To exclude ... I would do ...

- Rule out medical diagnoses and organic causes or other functional causes
- FBC, UE, Cr, TFT, glucose, LFT's, urinary drug screen, EEG, CT scan may show structural abnormalities, enlargement of the ventricular system (Johnstone and Andreasen) and prominent sulci-cortex
- MRI – cerebral blood flow and glucose utilization in the prefrontal cortex

- Collateral history and additional information from sources to find out ....
- Role of other professionals – to do what?

Establish a therapeutic alliance

Maximize collaborative approach to treatment. Understand patients attitude to medication and its importance for compliance.

DECREASE SYMPTOMS USING A BIOPSYCHOSOCIAL MODEL

Biological

- Decrease symptoms with neuroleptics, benzodiazepines, oral intramuscular /intravenous
- Choose medication by consideration of past treatment responses, side effect profile, patient preferences, route of administration
- Monitor compliance and side effects
- Consider high, intermediate and low potency antipsychotics
- Haloperidol 5–20mg, fluphenazine
- Chlorpromazine 300–1000 mg, thioridazine 100–600 mg
- Risperidone 4–6 mg (Range 2–8 mg/day)
- Olanzapine 10–20 mg (Range 5–20 mg/day: usually 10 mg/day)
- Sertindole 12–24 mg (Range 4–20 mg/day)
- Treat comorbid depression and anxiety or drug and alcohol withdrawal

Side effects

- Sedation – may be desirable
- Anticholinergic, e.g. dry mouth, blurred vision, constipation, tachycardia and urinary retention, antiadrenergic effects – hypotension
- Anticholinergic toxicity – impaired memory, cognition, confusion, delirium, somnolence and hallucinations
- Extrapyramidal side effects – acute, Parkinsonism, dystonia, akathisia, neuroleptic malignant syndrome, tardive dsykinesia – see chapter 11.1 on movement disorders
- Seizures
- Endocrine effects – galactorrhoea and oligomenorrhoea
- Weight gain
- Sexual dysfunction
- Allergic and hepatic effects
- Opthalmological effects
- Haematological effects

Psychological

- Psychoeducation to patients and carers
- Develop therapeutic alliance
- Transference/counter transference
- Reassurance/support
- Decrease stimulation by one-to-one interactions, small unit, stimulus decreasing strategies if acute, clear practical goals

- Chronic patients need structured organized environment
- Decrease over stimulation or stressful life events
- Treat comorbid substance dependence with education, harm reduction, abstinence, relapse prevention and rehabilitation

Social

- Assemble supports, finance, housing, family, nursing staff, issues
- Develop plan for continuing treatment

SHORT-TERM MANAGEMENT

Safety

Decrease symptoms using a biopsychosocial approach

Biological

- Antipsychotic medication – restore level of functioning
- Monitor side effects and compliance, consider depot

Psychological

- Therapeutic alliance with family and patient
- Cognitive behavioural therapy – anxiety, social skills training, delusions, hallucinations, problem solving, communication skills
- Supportive psychotherapy: patient, family

Social

- Advocacy, practical assistance – house, money, family support, nursing staff, social skills, maintain independence
- Social skills training

LONG-TERM MANAGEMENT

Safety

Decrease symptoms using a biopsychosocial approach

Biological

- Optimal treatment, consider treatment resistance, e.g. dose, side effects, compliance, adjunct treatment, clozapine, risperidone – antagonist activity at the serotonin type 2 receptors and at the dopamine type 2 receptor. Associated with fewer neurological side effects

Clozapine – weak antagonist of D2 receptor but appears to be an antagonist of the D4 receptor and antagonistic activity at the serotonergic receptors and antihistaminergic
- Prior to start make sure medical history taken as seizures will exclude use
- Baseline FBC and informed consent. Test dose of 25–50 mg, early side effects – severe hypotension. As tolerance develops to side effects increase to 200–600 mg/day (range). Monitor blood weekly WBC, risk of agranulocytosis if <3000 mm³.
- *Side effects*
    — Central nervous system – drowsy, fits, tremor, akathisia
    — Autonomic nervous system – dry mouth, sweat, hypersalivation
    — Cardiovascular – tachycardia, post ECG change
    — Gastrointestinal – nausea, vomiting, constipation, weight gain
    — Miscellaneous – granulocytopenia, rash, hypothermia, eosinophilia
- Effective in 30–60% of treatment resistant patients, decreases negative symptoms, little tardive dyskinesia
- Clozapine trial should last at least 3 months at 200–600 mg/day

Risperidone – a benzisoxamide
- *Side effects* – postural hypotension, sedation, weight gain, insomnia, fatigue, blurred vision, Dose range 1-8 mg/day: 1-2 mg/day usually for first episode psychosis or elderly patients: chronic patients usually require 2-8 mg/day.

Olanzapine – 2-methyl-4-(4methyl-1-piperazinyl)-10H-thienol[2,3][1,5]benzodiazepine. Range 5–20 mg/day: usually 10 mg/day
- *Side effects* – somnolence and weight gain, occasional dizziness, increased appetite, peripheral oedema, orthostatic hypotension and mild transient anticholinergic effects, rare – photosensitivity, hyperprolactineaemia, occasional elevation of LFTs,

Sertindole – 4 mg/day and increase by 4 mg every 2–3 days
- *Side effects* – orthostatic hypotension, mild increase in prolactin levels, rhinitis, decrease ejaculatory volume in men, increase in QT interval on ECG. Dosage 5–10 mg/day as a single dose, increase to >10 mg/day only after clinical review (5–20 mg/day)

Depot treatment useful in non-compliance.
- Flupenthixol decanoate: 40 mg every 2 weeks
- Zuclopenthixol decanoate: 200 mg every 2 weeks
- Haloperidol decanoate: 100 mg every 4 weeks
- Fluphenazine decanoate: 25 mg every 2 weeks
- Risk of tardive dyskinesia, neuroleptic malignant syndrome
- Know doses of chlorpromazine equivalents
    100 mg chlorpromazine = 12.5 mg fluphenazine every 3 weeks = 30 mg haloperidol decanoate every month
    100 mg chlorpromazine = 5 mg trifluoperazine = 2 mg haloperidol = 2 mg pimozide = 100 mg clozapine = 1 mg risperidone

Other issues:

- Marder (1987) looked at the amount of fluphenazine and tried 5 and 25 mg over 2 years: concluded that 25 mg better
- Cole and Davis – medication superior to placebo
- Rifkin – medication (fluphenazine) superior to placebo
- Decrease in dose will increase symptoms and relapse potential
- Decrease in dose will decrease extrapyramidal side effects (Kane, Marder, Johnstone, Hogarty)

- Geriatric patients – start on high potency agents as these cause less hypotension and therefore reduce the risk of falls. They are also less cholinergic (less likely to cause delirium, constipation and urinary retention) and less sedative (less likely to cause agitation). Consider use of risperidone

Lithium to augment the antipsychotic response especially if also affective symptoms

- Usually added to antipsychotic medication after patient had an adequate trial and has reached a plateau in level of response. Need level of 0.8–1.2 m eq./litre
- Response to treatment appears promptly

Psychological

- Foster therapeutic alliance
- Cognitive behavioural techniques – patient, family – problem solving techniques, communication
- Decrease expressed emotion in families
- Psychoeducation of individual, encourage blame free acceptance of illness and strategies to promote control of the illness
- Communication training
- Problem solving training
- Relapse prevention
- Compliance management
- Reinforcement of personal boundaries

Common components in successful intervention (Lam 1991):

- Positive approach, establish working relationship with family
- Provide structure and stability
- Focus on 'here and now' – strengths and weakness of coping
- Use 'family system' concepts – boundaries, coalitions, triangulation
- Cognitive techniques re unhelpful attributions, e.g. guilt
- Behavioural approaches – goal setting, problem solving

Social

- Case manager, housing, finances, vocation, retrain, liaise with employer rehabilitate
- Avoid over or under stimulation
- Aims: prevent clinical impairment; reduce social disadvantage; improve self confidence and self help skills
- Assertive outreach if patient does not attend for appointments etc or is non compliant – use phone calls, home visits
- Organized support groups

DISCUSSION ISSUES

EPIDEMIOLOGY

- 15–20 per 100,000 per year
- Prevalence 0.5–1%

- Lifetime risk – 0.9%
- Median age of onset – 28 males, 32 females
- Increased prevalence in lower social class – social drift, but may be more stresses associated with social class IV and V
- Increased perinatal injuries
- Increased left handedness
- Increase in winter births
- Increased incidence of low birth order if from a large family

FAMILY PROCESSES

- High frequency of life events in 3 weeks before a relapse
- Relapse rate increases:
    — If family shows high expressed emotion (critical comments or over involvement at a standardized interview)
    — More than 35 hours per week is spent in high expressed emotion environment
    — Not taking neuroleptics
- The assessment of expressed emotion involves analysing the content of what is said and the manner in which it is said
- Social intervention and training the family to reduce expressed emotion are therapeutically effective
- Psychosocial approaches show reduced relapse rates:
  Family interventions (Lam 1991)
  Early intervention (Birchwood and Shepher 1992)
  Coping strategies (Tanner 1993)
  Training in illness self management (Eckman et al. 1992)
- Hogarty looked at medication versus social skills training and family therapy. Found that least relapse if medication + social skills + family therapy
- Falloon, Tarrier and Hogarty show advantages of family therapy

SOCIAL PROCESSES

- Increased incidence of schizophrenia in inner city areas – Chicago
- Male schizophrenia shows low social class distribution
- Paternal occupations on birth certificates show normal social class distribution
- Social drift hypothesis – people with schizophrenia drift down the social scale
- Poverty of environment has been shown to be important. An increase in stimuli can diminish negative symptoms

NEUROLOGICAL ABNORMALITIES

- Increased ventricular size and other abnormalities on CT
- Age disorientation, impaired frontotemporal functioning, dysphasia

- Soft neurological signs, e.g. dygraphaesthesia, gait abnormalities, astereognosis, clumsiness found in many chronic schizophrenics even if they have very little physical or drug treatment

NEGATIVE SYMPTOMS

- Social isolation
- Poverty of thought or speech
- Lack of motivation, volition
- Affective flattening
- Inability to feel pleasure
- Impairment of attention and cognitive processes

PROGNOSIS

5 YEAR PROGNOSIS (with treatment)

- 55% chronic
- 45% acute improving course
- 49 % self supporting
- 11% chronic hospitalization

POOR PROGNOSIS

- Early onset
- Insidious onset
- Lack of precipitants
- Disorganized symptoms
- Lack of affective component
- Low IQ
- Low social class
- Abnormal premorbid personality
- Negative symptoms
- Neurological signs and symptoms
- Perinatal trauma
- No remissions in 3 years
- Relapses
- History of assaultiveness
- Family history of Schizophrenia
- Social isolation

Prognosis is affected by:

- Degree of effective family or other support available and used
- Attractiveness of the person and personality, e.g. to an employer, spouse, health worker
- Useful skills which have been acquired
- Degree of intelligence, aptitude and willingness to work
- Compliance with treatment regimen

GOOD PROGNOSIS

- Late onset
- Precipitants
- Acute onset
- Good premorbid social, sexual, work histories
- Mood disorder symptoms
- Preservation of affect during acute episode
- Married
- Family history of mood disorders
- Good support systems
- Positive symptoms

GOOD PROGNOSIS FOR SCHIZOPHRENIFORM DISORDER

- Onset of psychosis in four weeks and a change of behaviour
- Confusion and perplexity at the height of the psychotic episode
- Good premorbid social and occupational functioning
- Absence of blunt or flat affect

GOOD PROGNOSTIC FEATURES FOR BRIEF PSYCHOTIC EPISODE

- Good premorbid adjustment
- Few schizoid traits
- Precipitating stressor is severe
- Affective symptoms
- Confusion and perplexity during psychosis
- Little affective blunting
- Short duration of symptoms
- Absence of relatives with schizophrenia

RISK FACTORS FOR SUICIDE IN SCHIZOPHRENIA

- Male
- Recent in-patient discharge
- Unemployed
- Young
- Chronic illness
- Depression
- High premorbid educational achievement
- Lives alone

Additional risk factors include:

- Suicidal ideas, command auditory hallucinations to kill oneself and recent discharge from hospital
- 10–15% commit suicide

- Monitor closely patients during times of personal crisis, significant environmental changes or heightened distress or depression during the course of the illness

POST PSYCHOTIC DEPRESSION

Common:

- Increased risk compared with the general population
- 60% have a depressive episode sometime in course of the illness
- 50% of the patients recovering from acute illness and 25 % of those in remission
- Post-psychotic depression is associated with poor outcome, increased suicide, impaired work and social performance, and an increased risk of relapse and longer hospitalizations
- Post-psychotic depression is distinguished from major depression by the absence of mood disorder in first-degree relatives, stability of schizophrenic diagnosis and response to antipsychotic rather than antidepressant drugs
- Treat with SSRIs, lithium, tricyclic antidepressants

VIOLENT BEHAVIOUR

Risk factors include:

- Arrests
- Substance abuse
- Hallucinations
- Delusions
- Bizarre Behaviour
- Neurological impairment
- Male
- Unskilled
- Uneducated
- Unmarried
- Poverty

May need to sedate and use restraint and seclusion, and consider use of midazolam and droperidol or zuclopenthixol acetate (50–150mg)

Psychosis-induced polydipsia

- Compulsive water drinking associated with psychological disturbances and hyponatremia occurs in 6–20% of patients with chronic mental illnesses
- Exclude medical causes, e.g. diabetes mellitus, insipidus, chronic renal failure, hypocalcaemia and hypokalaemia
- Manage by water restriction and sodium replacement to prevent seizures and consequences of hyponatraemia. Control psychosis and water intake. May need lithium and phenytoin

Type I and Type II (Crow 1980)

- Type I symptoms respond to antipsychotic, positive symptoms – possible increase in dopamine receptors
- Type II symptoms less responsive to medication, negative symptoms? Cell loss and structural changes in the brain

TREATMENT COMPLIANCE

The degree to which the patient carries out the clinical recommendations of the treating physician. Level of non-compliance is high in discharged patients with schizophrenia, 50% after 1 year and 75% after 2 years have been reported to be non-compliant post-discharge (Weiden *et al.* 1994). Examples of compliance include keeping appointments, taking medication correctly, entering a treatment programme, following specific recommendations. Consider the following factors:

- Patient factors
- Drugs
- Prescriber

Patient factors

- Denial
- Drugs – fear effects and stigma, altered lifestyle
- See medication as a 'moral weakness'
- Feel immunity to medicine
- Can't understand regime
- Loss of comfort of hallucinations – left 'empty' if long standing hallucinations are cured – need to help patients regain occupational and leisure skills
- Disappearance of manic feelings
- Medication continues to remind them of illness
- Sick role diminishes
- Psychosocial – poor social support, carers antagonistic to medication
- Attitudinal – hostility to authority, delusional beliefs about medication
- Lack of insight
- Disempowerment

Drugs

- No immediate deterioration when stop drugs
- Complex regime
- Treatment variables – complexity, side effects

Prescriber

- Complex regime
- Poor communication
- Doctor-patient relationship – patient dissatisfaction, attitude to medication of the therapist

Improve compliance by:

- Attitude to illness and medicine of patient
- Enthusiasm of physician
- Decrease waiting times
- Time spent talking to patient and explaining treatment
- Least difficult schedule, once daily instead of three times a day
- Name of medication is explained and the side effects
- Dosage dispensed regularly
- Awareness of patients belief system, enlist patient help in establishing treatment regime
- Develop collaborative therapeutic relationship

COMMUNITY TREATMENT ORDERS

Discuss their usefulness and indications for. What are the procedures if they remain non compliant?

CASE MANAGEMENT

Enables the person to have one key worker who takes responsibility for their overall management using a biopsychosocial model.

TREATMENT RESISTANCE

- Review diagnosis
- Observe drug free if possible
- Check compliance
- Increase dose
- Use another drug from a different class
- Add an adjunct
- What other issues are contributing to maintaining symptoms, e.g. psychological, social
- Use of other treatments, e.g. group, cognitive behavioural therapy, social skills training

TREATMENT FOR SCHIZOAFFECTIVE DISORDER

Schizoaffective disorder has a better prognosis than schizophrenia and a worse prognosis than mood disorder.

DEFINITIONS OF THOUGHT PROCESS

Know progression from normal, circumstantial (reach goal), tangential (answer question at a tangent, will not reach goal), flight of ideas (connections can be followed), loosening of associations or derailment (illogical connections, cannot follow), word salad (incoherent).

FIRST RANK SYMPTOMS OF SCHIZOPHRENIA

- Thought insertion, broadcast, withdrawal
- Somatic hallucinations
- Made acts, impulses, affect, i.e. passivity
- Audible thoughts, voices arguing about the subject (*Gedankenlautwerden*)
- Voices commenting on the actions of the third person
- Delusional perception

PRINICIPLES OF REHABILITATION

See chapter 7.1

MOVEMENT DISORDERS

See chapter 11.1

ABNORMAL INVOLUNTARY MOVEMENT SCALE

- Either before or after completing the examination procedure, observe the patient unobtrusively at rest
- The chair to be used in this examination is a hard, firm one without arms
- After observing to patient rate him or her on a scale of 0 (none),1 minimal, 2 (mild), 3 (moderate) and 4 (severe) according to the severity of symptoms
- Ask the patient whether there is anything in his or her mouth, e.g. gum and if so to remove it
- Ask the patient about the current condition of his or her teeth. Ask if he or she wears dentures. Do teeth or dentures bother the patient now?
- Ask patient whether he or she notices any movement in mouth, face, hands or feet. If yes, ask patient to describe and indicate to what extent they currently bother patient or interfere with his or her activities
- Have the patient sit in chair with hands on knees, legs slightly apart and feet flat on the floor (look at entire body for movements while in this position)
- Ask patient to sit with hands hanging unsupported. If male, between legs, if female and wearing a dress, hanging over knees. Observe hands and other body areas
- Ask patient to open mouth. Observe tongue at rest within mouth. Do this twice
- Ask the patient to protrude tongue. Observe abnormalities of tongue movement. Do this twice
- Ask the patient to tap thumb, with each finger, as rapidly as possible for 10–15 seconds, separately with right hand, then with left hand. Observe facial and leg movements
- Flex and extend patient's left and right arms (one at a time)
- Ask patient to extend both arms outstretched in front with palms down. Observe trunk, legs and mouth

2.3 SCHIZOPHRENIA CASE

IDENTIFICATION

34-year-old man, divorced, currently on an invalid pension.

ISSUES

Management of a relapse of schizophrenic illness.

DIFFICULTIES

Poor historian.

PRESENTING COMPLAINT

- 'Very sick and feels tired'
- Referred by case manager. Has recently had an increase in medication (clozapine) from 200 to 300 mg bd

HISTORY OF PRESENTING COMPLAINT

- Three days ago started hearing voices that comment on his actions, e.g. 'he is lying in bed ...' and also hears his boss talk about him with other voices "millions". The voices do not tell him to perform any actions
- He thinks that the television talks about him and also that someone is trying to kill him as the result of him working last year in a shop. He witnessed occasional illicit transactions and now thinks that because he knows 'too much' he is in danger. He believes that people in the street talk about him

PAST PSYCHIATRIC HISTORY

- 1980 – admitted to hospital hearing voices? What treatment?
- 1982 – year long admission treated with chlorpromazine
- 1985 – 3-month admission treated with trifluoperazine and chlorpromazine
- 1990 – admission – treated with trifluoperazine
- 1994 – treated with clozapine

RELEVANT NEGATIVES

- He has had some sleep disturbance, no early morning wakening, energy levels are poor, he is able to concentrate, no suicidal ideation or intent. He is tearful on occasion but does not feel guilty. He is not homicidal
- He drinks occasionally but not since last year. Used to drink seven schooners a day and whisky, and would experience blackouts. He has not experienced head injuries, delirium tremens or fits. Has used marijuana prior to his first admission but nil since

CONSEQUENCES

Currently unable to work, spends days lying in bed, isolated and alone.

MANAGEMENT SO FAR

Wants to go back to using trifluoperazine which he was on for 11 years. He hears voices when he's out of hospital. Has been seeing case manager but stopped 2 months ago.

CURRENT TREATMENT

On clozapine medication 300 mg bd. Dislikes this due to the blood tests.

FAMILY HISTORY

Grandmother committed suicide in 1980 and used to hear voices.

PERSONAL HISTORY

Born in England, brought as a young child to Australia as parents migrated in search of a better life. Parents worked hard in their own business and so was brought up by a housekeeper whom he describes as 'cruel' and 'uncaring'. He studied hard and did well at school, and on leaving had various clerical jobs.

He was married and has a child. The marriage split up due to his drinking. He was not violent. Since 1990 he has been on a pension and living in a hostel. His contact with his family is poor and he describes himself as lonely.

CIGARETTES

Smokes one pack a day.

FORENSIC

Nil.

PREMORBID PERSONALITY

Enjoys reading and music. Has no friends and feels depressed.

MENTAL STATE EXAMINATION

- Appearance and behaviour – casually dressed, cooperative, no abnormal mannerisms or movements
- Speech was tangential at times, i.e. would answer a question with an unrelated answer
- Mood was depressed, scared and worried
- Affect was frightened and perplexed and dysphoric with little mobility
- No suicidal ideation or intent
- Thought content was preoccupied with being hurt by someone as a result of knowing too much, i.e. delusions of persecution, also delusions of reference in that he believed the TV and radio were talking about him
- No disorder of thought possession
- Experiences auditory hallucinations which discuss him and comment on his actions
- Cognition – mini mental state score was 27/30 with the abnormalities being on short-term memory testing
- Insight – did not think he was ill but would accept medication

ON EXAMINATION

Exclude any extrapyramidal side effects, stigmata of alcohol abuse, endocrine abnormalities.

SUMMARY

In conclusion a 31-year-old man, divorced, who was admitted following an exacerbation of auditory hallucinations and persecutory delusions. He is having side effects from an increase of dosage of clozapine, which has left him feeling drowsy while increasing his weight and appetite. He has a history of multiple admissions to hospital and there is a genetic predisposition for schizophrenia. He is socially isolated in that he has few friends. His marriage broke up 8 years ago. He has a history of casual jobs over the years with occupational decline. He used to use alcohol as a way of coping with the auditory hallucinations. Currently he has perplexed and dysphoric affect, delusions of reference and experiences auditory hallucinations commenting on him and discussing him.

His admission appears to be precipitated by alteration in medication. He is compliant with medication although he feels it is not working. He initiated admission via his case worker which shows some insight into his condition. He spends most of the day alone and this may be to protect himself from interacting with others with alcohol problems. His personal safety is of paramount importance as he is currently feeling hopeless about the situation and persecuted by voices.

DIAGNOSIS

Paranoid schizophrenia.

ISSUES FOR DISCUSSION

- Differential diagnosis
- Role of depression in schizophrenia
- Dangerousness
- Risk to self
- Social aspects, e.g. accommodation
- Comorbidity e.g. substance use/alcohol
- Treatment resistance

2.4 PARANOID PATIENT

IDENTIFICATION

Female > male, age 40–55 years.

CULTURE

?Delusional in this culture, prevalence 0.03%, lifetime morbidity risk of 0.05–0.1 %.

ISSUES

Safety, clarify diagnosis, management and compliance.

DIFFICULTIES

Hostility, veracity, denial.

REFERRAL

Friends, relatives, police, courts, neighbours.

PRESENTING COMPLAINT

Problems, harassment of others.

HISTORY PRESENTING COMPLAINT

Symptoms: systematized delusions, paranoid, persecutory, somatic hypochondriasis, hallucinations.

DELUSIONAL DISORDER

Use mnemonic *NOAR*

*N*on bizarre delusions
not *O*bviously bizarre behaviour
*A*uditory hallucinations, not prominent
*R*ule out affective, schizophrenia and organic

DIAGNOSTIC CRITERIA FOR DELUSIONAL DISORDER Modified with permission from the
Diagnostic and Statistical Manual of Mental Disorders, Fourth Edition. Copyright 1994 American Psychiatric Association.

- Non-bizarre delusions (i.e. involving situations that occur in real life such as being followed, poisoned, infected, loved at a distance, or deceived by spouse or lover, or having a disease) of at least 1-month duration
- Criteria A for Schizophrenia have never been met (Note: tactile and olfactory hallucinations may be present in delusional disorder if they are related to the delusional theme)
- Apart from the impact of the delusion(s) or its ramifications, functioning is not markedly impaired and behaviour is not obviously odd or bizarre
- If mood episodes have occurred concurrently with delusions their total duration has been brief to the duration of the delusional periods
- The disturbance is not due to the direct physiological effects of a substance or general medical condition (e.g. a drug of abuse, a medication) or a general medical condition

Specify type:

- Erotomania: delusions that another person, usually of higher status, is in love with the individual
- Grandiose: delusions of inflated worth, power, knowledge, identity or special relationship to a deity or famous person
- Jealous type: delusions that the individuals sexual partner is unfaithful
- Persecutory type: delusions that the person (or someone to whom the person is close) is being malevolently treated in some way
- Somatic type: delusions that the person has some physical defect or general medical condition
- Mixed type: delusions characteristic of more than one of the above types but no one theme predominates
- Unspecified type

Paranoid delusions can be part of formal psychiatric illness or paranoid states

ONSET

Course is insidious, may be precipitated by breakdown, migration.

CONSEQUENCES OF SYMPTOMS

- Psychiatric – suicidal, homicidal
- Social – relationship and forensic activities
- Physical – refusal to eat or drink

TREATMENT AND MANAGEMENT SO FAR

Response and compliance.

RELEVANT NEGATIVES

Schizophrenia, drugs and alcohol, suicidal, homicidal.

SEVERITY

Disruption to lifestyle, and dangerousness

COMORBIDITY

Depression, drugs and alcohol, obsessive compulsive disorder, body dysmorphic disorder, paranoid, schizoid, avoidant personality disorders

FAMILY HISTORY

- More common in relatives of individuals with schizophrenia
- Avoidant and paranoid personality disorder may be especially common among first-degree relatives of individuals with delusional disorder

PERSONAL HISTORY

- Post or prenatal insult, early environment was hostile, dangerous, basic trust did not develop, parental relationship and relationship with siblings, abuse, loss, discord, school achievements; relative quality and duration, occupation, change in functioning, isolated and has problems with colleagues and employers
- Life event losses, diagnosis, migration, deaths, social, family loss, isolation, loneliness

FORENSIC

Litigation, assault, damage, police, restraining orders, charges convictions.

PAST PSYCHIATRIC HISTORY

Chronicity, fluctuations, past treatment and response outcome, past dangerousness.

PAST MEDICAL HISTORY

Head injury, cerebral insult, cardiovascular, drug and alcohol, HIV.

PREMORBID PERSONALITY

- Isolated, self esteem decreased, hypersensitive to criticism, hostile and angry
- Schizoid, paranoid, avoidant traits, eccentric
- Dynamics – denial, reaction formation, not accept ideas, splitting, projection

DRUGS AND ALCOHOL

Morbid jealousy, amphetamines – paranoid psychosis.

MENTAL STATE

Poor eye contact, rapport, suspicious, anxiety, agitated, irritable, depressed, homicidal, systematized delusions, not prominent hallucinations, cognition intact.

ON EXAMINATION

Increased arousal, drugs and alcohol, central nervous system, cardiovascular disease.

DIFFERENTIAL DIAGNOSIS OF DELUSIONAL DISORDER

- Delirium
- Dementia
- Psychotic disorder due to a general medical condition*
- Substance-induced psychotic disorder
- Schizophrenia and schizophreniform – absence of any other symptoms of the active phase of Schizophrenia, more impairment with schizophrenia
- Mood disorder with psychotic features
- Psychotic disorder not otherwise specified
- Hypochondriasis
- Body dysmorphic disorder
- OCD
- Paranoid personality disorder   *see over*

*Psychotic disorder due to general medical condition

- Neurological, e.g. neoplasms, cerebrovascular disease, Huntington's disease, epilepsy, auditory nerve injury, deafness, migraine, CNS infections, Alzheimer's, multiple sclerosis, multi-infarct dementia
- Endocrine, e.g. hyper- and hypothyroidism, hyper- and hypoparathyroidism, hypoadrenocorticism
- Metabolic, e.g. hypoxia, hypercarbia, hypoglycaemia, fluid or electrolyte imbalances, hepatic or renal disease
- Autoimmune, e.g. systemic lupus erythematosus

Delusions more common if temporal lobe is affected or central nervous system

Risk factors – paranoid, avoidant, schizoid personality disorder

Life events stresses, immigration, deafness, loss of support system and decline in socio-economic status

MANAGEMENT

Safety

Dangerous, treat, assault, past violence, humiliation, fear revenge.

Clarify diagnosis

- Observations and disability
- Exclude differential diagnosis

SPECIAL INVESTIGATIONS

To exclude ... I would do ...

FBC, UE, TFT, glucose, B_{12}, folate, ESR, LFT, Ca, PO_4, VDRL, HIV, CXR, ECG, CT/MRI, neuropsychological testing.

- Collateral history to provide additional information
- Role of other professionals – to do what? Occupational therapist, assess activities of daily living, home visit, support, life events

Establish a therapeutic alliance

Decrease symptoms using a biopsychosocial model

Biological

Low dose of antipsychotics, e.g. pimozide 2 mg bd (increase by 2 mg to a maximum of 20 mg), trifluoperazine 5–10 mg, haloperidol 2–15 mg/day.

Treat comorbid depression

Psychosocial

- Empathic listening, do not collude, non confrontation
- Coping styles and hypersensitivity

Social

Life stresses, advocacy.

LONG-TERM MANAGEMENT

Inpatient

- Rehabilitation approach, accommodation, isolation, employment, advocacy, case management, monitor regularly, depression, sensory input
- Dangerousness
- Psychosocial – relationships
- Do not collude, gently challenge

Aetiology

- Recent theories that delusions are a defence against depression. Munro used pimozide and an antidepressant to relieve both delusions and depression – of 49 patients with pimozide eight developed depression. When pimozide withdrawn then depression subsided and delusions returned
- Review by Zigler and Glick – argue delusions are defensive process to ward off depression, paranoid symptoms in schizophrenia and manic in bipolar affective disorder

EATING DISORDERS

3.1 ANOREXIA NERVOSA

IDENTIFICATION

Age, female, school, culture.

ISSUES

- Chronic illness, early onset, development, morbidity
- Management problems

DIFFICULTIES

Minimization, hostility, denial, collusion by parents with patient, presentation of 'false self' by patient.

REFERRAL

Self, relatives, police, deliberate self harm, liaison.

HISTORY OF PRESENTING COMPLAINT

Use mnemonic *RABID*

*R*efusal to maintain weight - 15%
*A*menorrhoea
*B*ehaviours - weight losing behaviours
*I*ntense morbid fear of further weight gain
*D*isturbance in the way weight and size are perceived

DIAGNOSTIC CRITERIA FOR ANOREXIA NERVOSA Modified with permission from the Diagnostic and Statistical Manual of Mental Disorders, Fourth Edition. Copyright 1994 American Psychiatric Association.

- Refusal to maintain body weight at or above a minimally normal weight for age and height (e.g. weight loss leading to maintenance of body weight less than 85% of that expected: or failure to make expected weight gain during period of growth, leading to body weight less than 85% of that expected)
- Intense fear of gaining weight or becoming fat, even though underweight
- Disturbance in the way in which ones body weight or shape is experienced, undue influence of body weight or shape on self evaluation or denial of the seriousness of the current low body weight
- In postmenarcheal females, amenorrhoea, i.e. the absence of at least three consecutive menstrual cycles (a woman is considered to have amenorrhoea if her periods occur only following hormone, e.g. oestrogen administration)

Specify if:

Restricting type

Binge eating/purging

- Exact nature of problem as seen by patient - onset and course
- Attitude to shape, weight, decrease and increase to desired shape
- Intense fear of weight gain, body size and shape
- Eating habits - meals, amount, type, range, chronological, skip meals, restrict calories, hoard, hiding and bingeing
- Methods, vomit, purge, exercise, diuretic, diet pills
- Behaviour with food, e.g. cut food into small pieces and fat avoidance
- Precipitants- family, school, medical illness, relations and life events, bereavement, glandular fever, diet with peers
- Severity - maximum and minimum weight, physical condition and impairment of functioning
- Other behaviours include shoplifting, hoarding, compulsive shopping

CONSEQUENCES

- Physical - short of breath, palpitations, faint, weak, amenorrhoea
- Psychological - dependent, anxiety, sleep disturbance, apathy, decreased concentration and deliberate self harm
- Social - school, occupation, family, peers, relations, financial

TREATMENT TO DATE AND RESPONSE

RELEVANT NEGATIVES

Depression, psychosis, deliberate self harm, obsessive compulsive disorder (often comorbid but often not disclosed).

FAMILY HISTORY

- Psychiatric illness, eating problems, 7% siblings, depressed and anxious, deliberate self harm, drugs and alcohol, enmeshment, over protectiveness, rigidity, communication
- Increased risk of anorexia nervosa among first degree biological relatives of individuals with the disorder. Increased mood disturbances in relatives of patients with anorexia nervosa
- Monozygotic twins > dizygotic twins

PERSONAL HISTORY

Early development, sexual abuse, school, adolescence, psychosexual development.

PAST MEDICAL HISTORY

Physical illness in childhood.

PAST PSYCHIATRIC HISTORY

Eating disorder, depression 25-50%, anxiety, deliberate self harm, obsessional 20%.

SOCIAL

- Support of family/peers, finances, accomodation
- Family – enmeshment conflict and over-involvement

PREMORBID PERSONALITY

Borderline personality disorder

Use mnemonic *BIAS IRA*

Boredom
Identity
Anger
Suicide threats
Impulsivity
Relationships
Abandonment and affective instability

Obsessive compulsive personality disorder

Often has preoccupation with orderliness, perfectionism, mental and interpersonal control.

Low self esteem, perfect, obsessional.

MENTAL STATE EXAMINATION

- Often bright and alert, may be depressed, anxious, obsessive features and behaviour, body image, over valued ideas, suicidality
- Hunger is denied

ON EXAMINATION

Thin, peripheral cyanosis, lanugo hair, pubic and axillary hair, dry skin, cold extremities, hypotension, bradycardia, constipation, hyponatraemia, poor dentition, scarred knuckles, anaemia.

DIFFERENTIAL DIAGNOSIS

- General medical conditions, e.g. onset after the age of 40 years, GI disease, brain tumours, occult malignancies, AIDS, serious weight loss may occur
- Superior mesenteric artery syndrome characterised by postprandial vomiting secondary to intermittent gastric outlet obstruction
- Major depressive disorder
- Schizophrenia
- Social phobia
- Obsessive compulsive disorder
- Body dysmorphic disorder
- Bulimia nervosa
- Somatoform disorders
- Factitious
- Secondary gain
- Personality disorders
- Adjustment disorder

BULIMIA NERVOSA

Recurrent episodes of binge eating and inappropriate behaviour to avoid weight gain, e.g. self induced vomiting. Maintain body weight at a normal or minimally normal level - 50% of anorexia nervosa sufferers also meet criteria for bulimia nervosa.

Use mnemonic *BORCEN*

Binge - twice a week for 3 months
Over concern with body shape and image
Restricted eating or no eating between binges
Control of eating diminished
Engages in bulimic behaviour
Normal body weight

Age of onset for anorexia is 17 years, bimodal peak at 14 and 18 years. Rare over age 40. Mortality 10%.

MANAGEMENT ISSUES

- Safety and control
- Correct physical disturbance
- Treatment
- Restoration of eating patterns and prevention of relapse
- Family involvement and containment of parental anxiety
- Sibling rivalry, effect on siblings
- Disclosure of sexual, physical or emotional abuse
- Difficulties with developmental milestones, e.g. autonomy and identity
- Need for control and creativity expressed through thin body

Further assessment
Safety and dangerousness

- Psychological, suicidality, deliberate self harm, depression
- Physical - decrease K, Mg, PO_4, seizures, cardiac
- Secondary - weight loss, decreased heart size, bradycardia, arrhythmia

Clarify primary diagnosis

- Observations and disability
- Exclude differential diagnosis
- Collateral history to provide additional information
- Role of other professionals – to do what?
  Family dynamics, assessment, overprotectiveness, attitude, conflicts, dysfunction, Dietician, medical consults

Establish a therapeutic alliance

SPECIAL INVESTIGATIONS

To exclude ... I would do ...

Vital signs, FBC, UE, LFT, glucose, GGT, ESR, B_{12}, folate, Ca, PO_4, Mg, ECG, drug screen, 24 hour creatinine clearance, CT, DEXA.

DEXA

- Measures bone density in hips and spine
- <1 SD below age matched controls - osteopenia, 1 SD below - osteoporosis

Haematology

Leucopenia and mild anaemia are common, thrombocytopenia rarely.

Biochemistry

Dehydration increase blood urea nitrogen, hypercholesterolaemia, hypophosphataemia, hyperamylasemia, low oestrogen levels present in females and low testosterone levels in males, decreased T3, LH, FSH

ECG

Sinus bradycardia.

GIT

Delayed gastric emptying, bloating, constipation and abdominal pain.

EEG

Diffuse abnormalities and metabolic encephalopathy results from significant fluid and electrolyte disturbance.

Brain imaging

Increase in the ventricular-brain ratio secondary to starvation is often seen, brain regional blood flow abnormalities.

Pelvic ultrasound

Lack of ovulation, small ovaries

PHYSICAL SIGNS

- Signs often a result of starvation, abdominal pain, cold intolerance, lethargy, excess energy, emaciation, hypotension, dryness of skin, lanugo, bradycardia, peripheral oedema, yellowing of skin due to hypercarotenaemia, hypertrophy of the salivary glands and parotid glands
- Normochromic anaemia and impaired renal function and cardiovascular problems.
- Dental problems and osteoporosis, resulting from low calcium intake and absorption and reduced oestrogen secretion and increased cortisol secretion

- Hypoglycaemia, hypokalaemia, alkalosis
- May need opinion of cardiologist, endocrinologist

Treatment

- Refeeding - Electrolytes, urea, creatinine, blood sugar, ECG, weight gain, cardiac monitoring
- Correct imbalance
- If refeed rapidly may get a decrease in phosphate which may cause cardiac failure, shortness of breath and chest pain and delirium

Hospitalization is necessary if:

- Suicidal
- Rapid weight loss over 30% in 6 months
- Severe loss of energy
- Hypokalaemia < 3 meq/l or ECG changes despite K supplements
- Cycle of binge and vomiting cannot be broken
- Hypophosphataemia
- Dehydration
- Vomiting
- Psychosis

Hospital admission

- Bed rest with supervised feedings - frequent five to six meals are best and increase slowly from 1000 calories
- Initial intake is increased gradually so anorexics can select more food types
- Aim to refeed patient to Body Mass Index appropriate for age they become anorexic
- BMI = kg/m² Under 16 years BMI 18.5, > 16 years BMI 19+ depending on the premorbid weight or in patients < 16 years use percentile height and weight charts
- Weigh patient two to three times a week after urinating and before breakfast
- Attendant in bathroom or restrict access or bed rest for 2 hours after meals to prevent vomiting
- Positive reinforcement
- Forced feeding only if serious deterioration - nasogastric tube, dieticians, care with status, parental consent
- Education and nutritional information important for diet
- Set target weight of 90% and aim for increase of 1 kg per week
- Supervised eating and modelling
- Staff cohesion important and morale and burden - be aware of splitting by patients with team members. Need to deal with staff anxiety and counter transference
- Milieu important - multidisciplinary team, insight into behaviour
- Supervision of staff, need for firm leadership

Medicolegal issues

To treat or not to treat. Use Guardianship Act and occasionally Mental Health Act.

Pharmacotherapy

- Treat symptomatically, e.g. insomnia
- May need antidepressant, e.g. SSRI's
- Fluoxetine - 60 mg daily for bulimia nervosa
- Chlorpromazine if agitated or psychotic
- Oestrogen and Calcium therapy for osteoporosis

Psychotherapy

- Individual and group
- Supportive - contact, empathic listening, unconditional positive regard. More focused later, themes include control, weight gain, deficits in self esteem, autonomy
- Individual psychotherapy with family treatment
- Patients often present a 'false self' which is compliant
- Cognitive behavioural therapy - obsessions with being thin and low self esteem and tendency towards dichotomous thinking, e.g. fat versus thin, right versus wrong, cognitive distortions, automatic thoughts, inappropriate, self esteem and target weight
- Assertiveness skills, relaxation and social skills
- Family treatment - if admit, structural, dysfunctional family, anticipate difficulties, often problems with resistance, engagement and maintenance of treatment
- Discharge - target weight, monitor and week end leave, symptoms decrease, discharge plan, psychiatrist, dietician, group therapies

LONG-TERM MANAGEMENT

- Psychosocial - relapse prevention, bulimia, childbirth
- Chronic anorexia - palliative care
- Psychotherapy - individual, family, group, and self help
- Social advocacy - housing, welfare and vocational
- Prognosis - 20% symptomatic after 6 years. Mortality is 5-20% over 20 years and some develop a mood or phobic disorder
- CT scans show enlarged CSF spaces in anorexia nervosa patients during starvation, a finding that is reversed by weight gain

POOR OUTCOME

- Age at onset - late
- Continuously ill
- Disturbed relationships of patient and family
- Poor adjustment at school
- Low body weight on admission
- Osteoporosis
- Infertility
- Shortness of stature

AETIOLOGY

- Vulnerable personality
- Psychosocial conflicts
- Sociocultural factors
- Genetic and constitutional factors
- Female 10>male
- Sociocultural, family pathology, psychodynamic, psychobiological, obsessive compulsive disorder, constitutional development of difficulty and self esteem and pathogenic family, sexual abuse
- Weight phobia, low self esteem, parental conflict, hypothalamic disturbance
- Precipitants - stress, exams, dieting, illness, sexual, physical and emotional abuse, power issues
- Perpetuants - starvation factors, family, power, control and maintenance, ongoing abuse, power imbalance, domestic violence (subtle sometimes)

3.2 ANOREXIA NERVOSA CASE

IDENTIFICATION

June is a 15-year-old Caucasian girl living at home with her family and attending school. She is currently in hospital.

ISSUES

Management of anorexia nervosa in a 15-year-old.

DIFFICULTIES

Lack of acceptance of her condition.

REFERRED

Via her General Practitioner and parents 2 weeks ago.

PRESENTING COMPLAINT

'Anorexia'.

HISTORY OF PRESENTING COMPLAINT

- At the age of 12 years she started to diet and vomit by putting fingers down her throat. This lasted 3 months. When aged 14 she started to restrict her diet and increase exercise to lose weight. She did not abuse laxatives. She was eating daily two pieces of toast, cereal, rice and an apple at night. She was exercising daily and would weigh herself daily. Her periods stopped 1 year ago and she now weighs 43 kg. Her highest weight was 48 kg and her lowest weight 39 kg. At this time she started to binge on foods such as chocolate, chips, ice-cream, sausage, bread and would vomit after binges
- At the time of the first diet she wanted to look like a model and felt insecure with her friends and was having difficulties with parents over food

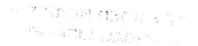

- She has lost 4 kg prior to admission despite being treated by the GP and psychiatrist. Her admission weight was 40 kg
- She is continuing her school work in hospital

RELEVANT NEGATIVES

She is not suicidal, does not abuse drugs or alcohol and there is no evidence of psychosis.

CONSEQUENCES

She thinks about food all the time and plans meals and events.

MANAGEMENT SO FAR

- She has been having a refeeding menu which consists of cereal, toast and an apple, sandwich, protein drink, hot meal of protein, carbohydrate and vegetables, tea, three biscuits, fruit, hot meal for dinner, dessert, supper of milk and two biscuits
- Current treatment includes bed rest after meals, refeeding, target weights, privileges, individual treatment, group therapy, dietician, psychologist, three times weekly weigh in, family therapy

FAMILY HISTORY

- Her parents are both teachers, she has an older brother and one younger sister. Her mother had a 'nervous breakdown' when June was aged 3 years
- She described her mother as strong willed and kind and her father as warm and sporty

PERSONAL HISTORY

- Born in the country, normal delivery and milestones
- Enjoys school and has good friends there. Started to become obsessive and moody about food at school and would refuse to eat with the family
- Her school grades were good and she was reported to be a good student
- She has had one boyfriend last year but has not had a sexual relationship
- She has worked in a supermarket

PAST MEDICAL HISTORY

No evidence of fits, epilepsy, faints, head injuries.

PAST PSYCHIATRIC HISTORY

She saw a psychologist a year ago and started a programme to control her eating and exercising.

ALCOHOL

She has drunk wine and spirits at parties and at home.

DRUGS

Does not use any.

CIGARETTES

Started smoking in hospital.

FORENSIC

Nil.

PREMORBID PERSONALITY

Friendly, open, enjoys piano playing, very neat with school work and has to tear things out if they do not reach the required standard.

MENTAL STATE EXAMINATION

- Appearance and behaviour - she is a very thin girl, dressed casually in track suit and trainers, wearing jewellery and make up. Appeared older than her stated years. She was cooperative and polite
- Her speech was coherent and spontaneous and there was no formal thought disorder.
- Her mood she described as 'up and down' adding she was tearful most days
- Her affect was euthymic, reactive and mobile. She was occasionally tearful when discussing family issues
- There was no suicidal ideation or intent
- Her thought content was mainly preoccupied with putting on weight as she was afraid that it would all turn to fat. She was worried that she would not be able to reach her target weight. She was also concerned about her family
- There was no disorder of thought possession and no abnormalities of perception elicited and she was not objectively hallucinating

- Cognitive testing proved unremarkable and she scored 30/30 on Mini Mental State Examination
- Insight - wants to eat however feels that she still has difficulties when eating food that contains fat
- Physical examination showed a bradycardia, blood pressure 90/50, cachectic, no lanugo hair, no parotid swelling, no oedema, no central nervous system abnormalities

SUMMARY

She is a 15-year-old admitted for management of anorexia nervosa. The problem started 3 years ago when she started dieting and vomiting. She started to diet again at the behest of a friend as she wished to look like a model. Now she is amenorrhoeic and afraid of becoming fat. There may be some family predisposition as her mother had a nervous breakdown. There have been difficulties within the family with food and many arguments. The problem first started when her sister was 2 years old. June was jealous of her and did not want another sibling. She is an eldest child and may be testing boundaries with the family by going out and drinking at parties. Her personality has some obsessive compulsive traits.

DISCUSSION ISSUES

- Diagnosis - anorexia nervosa
- Aetiology - hypothesise on family dynamics and meaning of symptoms
- Therapeutic alliance
- Relevance of premorbid personality
- Management issues - inside and outside hospital, follow up
- Role of family therapy

3.3 BULIMIA NERVOSA

IDENTIFICATION

Age (older than anorexic patient), female, marital status, living with, occupation, school, culture.

ISSUES

- Comorbidity, personality disorders, substance abuse, impulse control
- Physical consequences - purgative abuse, self harm

DIFFICULTIES

Hostility and denial.

REFERRAL

Self, family, school, emergency department, liaison and police.

HISTORY OF PRESENTING COMPLAINT

Use mnemonic *BORCEN*, and see chapter 3.2 on Anorexia Nervosa

*B*inge - twice a week for 3 months
*O*verconcern with body shape and image
*R*estricted Eating or no eating between binges
*C*ontrol of eating diminished
*E*ngages in bulimic behaviour
*N*ormal body weight

DIAGNOSTIC CRITERIA FOR BULIMIA NERVOSA Modified with permission from the Diagnostic and Statistical Manual of Mental Disorders, Fourth Edition. Copyright 1994 American Psychiatric Association.

A. Recurrent episodes of binge eating. An episode of binge eating is characterised by both of the following:

- Eating, in a discrete period of time (e.g. in any 2 hour period) an amount of food that is definitely larger than most people would eat during a similar period of time and under similar circumstances
- A sense of lack of control over eating during the episode, e.g. a feeling that one cannot stop eating or control what or how much one is eating

B. Recurrent inappropriate compensatory behaviour in order to prevent weight gain such as self induced vomiting, misuse of laxatives, diuretics, enemas, or other medications, fasting or excessive exercise.

C. The binge eating and inappropriate compensatory behaviour both occur, on average, twice a week for 3 months.

D. Self evaluation is unduly influenced by body shape and weight.

E. The disturbance does not occur exclusively during episodes of anorexia nervosa.

Specify if:

Purging type - during the current episode of bulimia nervosa the person has regularly engaged in self-induced vomiting or the misuse of laxatives, diuretics or enemas

Non-purging type - during the current episode of bulimia nervosa the person has used other inappropriate compensatory behaviours, such as fasting or excessive exercise, but has not regularly engaged in self-induced vomiting or the misuse of laxatives, diuretics or enemas

- Body weight is usually within 10% of normal
- Food habits and attitudes and beliefs
- Pattern of binge and vomit, weight loss and gain and menstrual history, typically carbohydrates sweet foods, e.g. ice cream and cakes
- Often binge when come home in the evenings
- Antecedents and behaviour and consequences
- Laxative, diuretics; amount and duration
- Comorbid - depression, anxiety, impulse control, substance abuse, shoplift, promiscuity, self harm, overspend, OCD, dysthymia
- Self image, evaluation of self and others

PRECIPITANTS

- Family, social, life event, developmental stage
- Severity - physical symptoms and impairment of function
- Loss, bereavement, change in life circumstances

CONSEQUENCES

- Physical - short of breath, alkalosis, anaemia, weak, osteoporosis, amenorrhoea, faint, poor dentition
- Psychological - self esteem, guilt, self harm
- Social and forensic - financial, occupational, school, family, peers, relations
- 80-90% of bulimics will vomit after a binge

FAMILY HISTORY

- Enmeshed care, controlled eating of food, eating problems, obesity
- Psychiatric illness - depression, anxiety, substance abuse
- History of sexual, emotional or physical abuse

PERSONAL HISTORY

- Early development, family relationships, abuse, separation, reflection, loss, school and peers, interpersonal relationship, psychosexual and adolescent development
- Often not living at home

PAST MEDICAL HISTORY

- Amenorrhoea, childhood illness, bulimia nervosa and consequences, e.g. gastric, inflammation, constipation, osteoporosis and renal
- Substance abuse: drug and alcohol sequelae

PAST PSYCHIATRIC HISTORY

Eating problem, e.g. anorexia, depression, anxiety, deliberate self harm, obsessive compulsive disorder, impulse control, shoplifting, gambling, substance abuse, compulsive abusive relationships.

PREMORBID PERSONALITY

Borderline personality disorder

Use mnemonic *BIAS IRA*

Boredom
Identity
Anger
Suicide threats
Impulsivity
Relationships
Abandonment and affective instability

Habit defences and ego strength, interpersonal relationships, mood and affect, self identity, self destructive behaviour, prone to anxiety, coping mechanisms, impulse control.

SOCIAL

- Support of family, peers, finances, accommodation
- Family: enmeshment, conflict, overinvolvement

FORENSIC

Nil.

MENTAL STATE EXAMINATION

Evidence of depression, anxiety, substance abuse, disturbance of body image, insight, cognitive disturbance and suicidality.

ON EXAMINATION

- Signs of anorexia or low weight, scarred knuckles, dentition, sexual and physical development, anaemia, constipation
- Enlarged parotid glands, menstrual irregularities
- Congestive cardiac failure, bradycardia, hypotension

DIFFERENTIAL DIAGNOSIS

- Anorexia nervosa - binge eating/purge type
- Central nervous system tumours
- Kleine-Levin syndrome - hypersomnia, hyperphagia
- Major depressive disorder with atypical features
- Borderline personality disorder
- Klüver-Bucy syndrome - visual agnosia, compulsive licking and biting, placidity, hypersexuality and hyperphagia
- Obsessive compulsive disorder
- Schizophrenia
- Bipolar affective disorder

MANAGEMENT

Safety and Dangerousness

- Suicidality, deliberate self harm, depression, forensic, impulsive behaviour

- Biological - physical electrolytes, alkalosis, cardiac arrthymias

Clarify diagnosis

- Observations re eating habits, exercise habits
- Exclude differential diagnosis

Comorbidity common with substance dependence

SPECIAL INVESTIGATIONS

To exclude ... I would do ...

FBC, UE, ESR, B_{12}, folate, Ca, glucose, PO_4, Mg, amylase, TFT, LH, FSH, oestradial, urinary drug screen, 24 hour creatinine clearance, ECG, CXR, CT, bone density.

- Collateral history to provide information on family dynamics, assessment
- Role of other professionals – to do what?

Medical complications

- Hypokalaemia, hypochloraemia, metabolic acidosis, hypoglycaemia
- Increased blood urea nitrogen
- Gastric rupture and tears
- Dental changes - loss of enamel, rounding of contours of the teeth and decalcification
- Painful swelling of the salivary glands

Establish a therapeutic alliance

Decrease symptoms and treat using biopsychosocial model

Biological

- Fluoxetine and other SSRI's
- Moclobemide/MAOI - atypical antidepressant
- Lithium and carbamazepine, beware self harm - use if comorbid mood disorders
- Alterations in thyroid and cortisol function
- Treat comorbid symptoms - often substance abuse

Psychosocial

Inpatient

- Restore eating patterns and nutritional rehabilitation, treatment and underlying psychological, social and family problems, prevent relapse and restore functioning
- Multimodal multidisciplinary team, dietician
- Treatment contract

Outpatient

- Motivated, social support, physically stable, not suicidal
- Multimodal model, correct physical problems, rapport and alliance, contract treatment
- Education - psychoeducation and nutritional
- Dietician assessment

Milieu, group

- Cognitive behavioural therapy - attitudes, shape, weight, affect, self esteem
- Group > individual

Behavioural

- Response prevention, planned meals three to five times a day to stop binge eating, diary, supervision, social skills, relaxation, decrease food in house, encourage exposure to forbidden foods
- Individual therapy - supportive, defences, here and now and empathic responses, confront and challenge, dynamic - conflict identity, interpersonal and family interpersonal
- Family treatment - education and problem solving, enlist support

LONG-TERM MANAGEMENT

Relapse prevention, rehabilitation, prevent consequences.

Biological

As above.

Psychological

- Individual and group, cognitive behavioural therapy
- Family
- Social advocacy - welfare, housing, financial
- Education for drugs, alcohol and treatment

Difficulties

Borderline personality disorder, drugs and alcohol, deliberate self harm, family, autonomy and denial.

Prognosis

- Outpatient - short-term, those who engage in treatment show 50% improvement in binge/purge, 80-90% decrease symptoms

- In-patient - poor outcome 33%, good 27%, one third some improvement to symptoms. Outcome not as well established although probably better than anorexia nervosa
- Some improvement with age

AETIOLOGY

- Biological - role of serotonin and noradrenaline
- Social - cultural pressure to be thin
- Psychological - use of own body as transitional object - ambivalence towards food, e.g. wish to fuse with the caretaker and regurgitating may express a wish for separation
- Use of bingeing and vomiting to deal with emotions, relationships and abuse

ANXIETY DISORDERS

4.1 ANXIETY

IDENTIFICATION

Age, sex, marital status, living with, occupation, culture.

ISSUES

Developmental stage, chronicity, comorbidity, impairment of functioning.

DIFFICULTIES

Anxiety, avoidance, embarassment.

REFERRED BY

Outpatient, liaison, self, family, employer, Emergency, General Practitioner, Social Services.

HISTORY OF PRESENTING COMPLAINT

- Anxiety disorders start in teens and early adulthood
- Psychological symptoms, fear, specific fears, apprehension, worry, depersonalisation, *feel unreal / strangely altered.* derealization, decreased concentration, insomnia, flashbacks, obsessions, compulsions
- Physiological symptoms – muscle tension, gastrointestinal tract, cardiovascular system, central nervous system, genitourinary system, autonomic system

1. Decide if the anxiety is pathological. Degree of secondary disability, handicap, decreased functioning.
2. Behavioural analysis ABC
   Antecedents
   Behaviour
   Consequences
   — Anticipatory anxiety
   — Avoidance
   — Avoid situations, problems at work, home
3. Precipitants to anxiety, e.g. in response to stress, adjustment reaction/bereavement.
4. Primary or secondary anxiety.
5. Related to drugs and alcohol.
6. Situational?

External versus Internal triggers

Panic	OCD, GAD (thoughts)
Phobias	Panic (sensations).
OCD (e.g. dirt)	

7. State versus trait.

COGNITIONS

- Establish the underlying cognition for the disorder
- Social phobia – fear of scrutiny, fear of embarrassment, fear of negative evaluation, fear of being the centre of attention
- Panic – fear of losing control
- Agoraphobia – fear of inability to escape, or help being unavailable
- GAD – fear of catastrophy or mistake
- OCD – specific obsession

DIFFERENTIAL DIAGNOSIS

- Primary anxiety disorder, e.g. generalised anxiety disorder, panic/agoraphobia, obsessive compulsive disorder, post traumatic stress disorder, specific phobia, social phobia
- Affective disorder, e.g. depression, agitation, dysthymia
- Somatoform, dissociative
- Schizophrenia – prodrome
- Personality disorder – especially avoidant, dependent
- Organic – stimulant abuse, caffeine, nicotine, sympathetic withdrawal, iatrogenic, thyrotoxicosis, phaeochromocytoma, Cushing's, hypoglycaemia, temporal lobe epilepsy, delirium, dementia
- Eating disorders
- B_{12} deficiency

Consider organic causes especially if first onset is after age 35 years

FAMILY HISTORY

Affective, anxiety, drugs and alcohol, suicide common.

PERSONAL HISTORY

- Childhood, parenting, separation, losses, abuses, rejection, discord, perinatal development, separation anxiety, school refusal, school performance, occupation, peers and interpersonal relationships, family and social support – primary and secondary gain
- Effect of disorder on occupation and social functioning

PAST MEDICAL HISTORY

Past illness as child, e.g. asthma. Current aetiology, endocrine, cardiovascular status, response to treatment outcome, sequelae of drugs and alcohol.

PAST PSYCHIATRIC HISTORY

Affective disorder, separation anxiety, school refusal, drugs and alcohol, deliberate self harm, treatment responses.

FORENSIC

Nil.

DRUG AND ALCOHOL HISTORY

- Alcohol and benzodiazepines
- Common – often comorbid with anxiety disorders
- *Ask why they take the substances*

PREMORBID PERSONALITY

Life long trait of anxiety, cluster C, dependent, avoidant, compulsion, timid, shy, fear of negative evaluation, social discomfort, submissive, difficulty making decisions, uncomfortable alone, strengths.

MENTAL STATE EXAMINATION

- Decreased eye contact, avoid gaze
- Affect, arousal and hypervigilance
- Behaviour – agitated, depressed, plaintive, psychotic
- Cognitive – themes, fear, apprehension, ruminations, obsessions, phobias

ON EXAMINATION

Pulse, temperature, blood pressure, autonomic over reactivity, sweating, goitre, Cushingoid, stigmata of drug and alcohol use.

MANAGEMENT

Safety, risk of suicide.

Clarify diagnosis

- Observations – assessment, severity, situational avoidance (this may be overt or subtle, e.g. avoid entirely or go only with company, change to life/way of living), anticipatory avoidance
- Exclude differential diagnosis
- Comorbid diagnoses e.g substance abuse, drugs + alcohol, may self medicate
- Avoidant personality disorder with social phobia will alter the type and amount of treatment required

---

SPECIAL INVESTIGATIONS

To exclude ... I would do ...

FBC, ESR, LFT, Ca, PO_4, TFT, Urinary VMA, CXR, ECG, EEG, CT.

Justify each test

- Collateral history and additional information from sources to find out ....
  Ask friends, doctors, family
- Role of other professionals – to do what?

Establish therapeutic alliance

Important to maximise compliance.

Decrease symptoms using a biopsychosocial model

Biological

- Identify precipitating and maintaining factors – caffeine, nicotine, alcohol
- Possibly a short course of benzodiazepines if severe
- Treatment – imipramine (classic along with MAOIs) – panic/agoraphobia
- Paroxitene, sertraline - panic disorder
- Clomipramine, fluvoxamine, fluoxetine, sertraline, paroxetine – obsessive compulsive disorder
- RIMAs/MAOIs – social phobia
- Antidepressants – GAD
- Treat comorbid depression, e.g. tricyclic antidepressants, monoamine oxidase inhibitors, selective serotonin reuptake inhibitors

Psychological

- Empathic listening, catharsis, support, instil hope, education, self help, development therapeutic alliance
- Foster internal locus of control – set reasonable goals
- Treatment of underlying cause if present
- Educate, feedback, handout
- Teach nature of anxiety and how it affects systems

- Relaxation technique, controlled breathing, instructions, tapes, set practise, hyperventilation model, increase insight
- Graded exposure
- Challenge irrational thoughts with rational ones – cognitive challenging
- Set homework

Social

Support, encouragement, cotherapist

LONG-TERM MANAGEMENT

Biological

Drugs, side effects, response, substance abuse, comorbid depression.

Psychosocial

- Rehabilitation, chronic issues
- Treatment depends on severity
- Simple intervention, education, psychological, drug and specialist centre or combination

GENERALISED ANXIETY DISORDER

IDENTIFICATION

- Male = female
- Come to attention in mid-20s but may not seek help until much later perhaps due to minimal interference with life
- Often present having felt anxious or nervous all their lives
- Describe themselves as 'worriers'
- Chronic course, fluctuates more in times of stress

HISTORY OF PRESENTING COMPLAINT

- Describes feelings of worry and tension most of the day, continuous thoughts playing in head, concerned about potential problems that may occur in the day
- Always worried and finding it hard to concentrate on work, feels tired and 'on edge'
- Worry is excessive and unreasonable and is understood as such by the patient
- Cognitive – function of worry – to prevent disaster
- Somatic symptoms
- Behavioural – avoid decisions

DIAGNOSTIC CRITERIA FOR GENERALISED ANXIETY DISORDER Modified with permission from the Diagnostic and Statistical Manual of Mental Disorders, Fourth Edition. Copyright 1994 American Psychiatric Association.

A. Excessive anxiety and worry (apprehensive expectation) occurring more days than not for at least 6 months about a number of events or activities (such as work or school performance).

B. The person finds it difficult to control the worry.

C. The anxiety and worry are associated with three (or more) of the following six symptoms (with at least some symptoms present for more days than not for the past 6 months).

- Feel restless, keyed up and on edge
- Being easily fatigued
- Difficulty concentrating or mind going blank
- Irritability
- Muscle tension
- Sleep disturbance – (difficulty falling and staying asleep or restless unsatisfying sleep)

D. The focus of anxiety and worry is not confined to axis 1 disorder, e.g. the anxiety or worry is not about having a panic attack (as in panic disorder), being embarrassed in public (as in social phobia), being contaminated (as in obsessive compulsive disorder), being away from home or close relatives (as in separation anxiety disorder), gaining weight (as in anorexia nervosa), having multiple physical complaints (as in somatization disorder) or having a serious physical illness (as in hypochondriasis) and the anxiety and worry do not occur exclusively during post traumatic stress disorder.

E. The anxiety, worry or physical symptoms cause clinically significant distress or impairment in social occupational or other important areas of functioning.

F. The disturbance is not due to the direct physiological effects of a substance (e.g. drug of abuse, a medication) or general medical condition (e.g. hyperthyroidism) and does not occur exclusively during a mood disorder, a psychotic disorder or a pervasive developmental disorder.

GAD

Use mnemonic *STOMACH*

Severity and vigilance
Two or more worries
Organic rule out
Motor tension
Anxiety unrelated
Course not psychotic
Hyper-reactive autonomic

RELEVANT NEGATIVES

Comorbidity with mood disorders (depression common), other anxiety disorders and substance dependence.

FAMILY HISTORY

Anxiety, depression.

PERSONAL HISTORY

- Possible emotional or verbal abuse, critical comments
- Anxiety disorders in family, may strive for perfection to avoid criticism, start to worry how to achieve goals
- Effect on occupation and relationships

DRUG AND ALCOHOL HISTORY

Often comorbid substance dependence.

PREMORBID PERSONALITY

Differs from 'worry' in the normal population as it is pervasive and lasts 6 months and causes interference with life and activities.

DIFFERENTIAL DIAGNOSIS

- Medical disorders which can cause anxiety – see chapter 4.2
- Exclude other anxiety disorders especially panic disorder and agoraphobia
- Exclude other axis I diagnoses, e.g. depression, dysthymia, substance dependence

TREATMENT

Individual or groups

Primary treatments are non pharmacological, e.g. exercise, sleep hygiene, relaxation – progressive muscular relaxation, cognitive behavioural therapy.

Cognitive behavioural therapy

- Five to 20 sessions
- Identify automatic thoughts, modify thoughts and associated behaviours, rationale, education, distraction
- Structured problem solving applied to worries – use as a treatment strategy
- Activity schedules, time management, reintroduction of pleasurable activities
- Verbal challenging of automatic thoughts and worries using cognitive behavioural techniques
- Questioning, looking for evidence, alternative explanations
- Exposure to avoided situation
- Social skills training, structured problem solving skills
- Self esteem – listing
- Use of flash cards
- Prevent relapse, decrease sessions, anticipate setbacks

Biological

Benzodiazepines

- These have been the biological treatment of choice. Try to use cognitive behavioural techniques rather than pharmacotherapy. Approximately 25–30% of patients fail to respond and tolerance and dependence may occur
- Think very carefully before initiating treatment
- The side effects include impaired cognitive performance, drowsiness, lethargy, and physical and psychological dependence with prolonged use
- Taper drug slowly. Do not continue treatment indefinitely.
- Discontinuation must be done carefully due to the possibility of a rebound anxiety or intensification of previous symptoms in others and risk of seizures
- Recommendations are for use in acute exacerbations, using a low dose and short time period
- The drugs may also have a mild disinhibiting action

Propranolol

- Sympathetic activity, subjective awareness
- Somatic anxiety e.g. peripheral symptoms, trembling, palpitations, restlessness, motor tension
- Dose 10–20 mg three or four times a day in divided doses, side effects: heart failure, conduction delay, asthma, depression, delirium psychosis, hypoglycaemia, diabetes

Buspirone – azaspirone

- Acts on 5-HT (serotonin) receptors
- Use in chronic anxiety and in patients with potential for substance abuse 20–30 mg in divided doses, >60 mg causes dysphoria
- Other side effects – headaches, dizziness, paradoxical excitement
- Effective in 60–80% of patients
- Produces no sedative effects or withdrawal symptoms or rebound anxiety following discontinuation

- May be suitable for long term use due to lack of dependence potential. Discontinuation can lead to resumption of original symptoms

Role of antidepressant medication if comorbid problem

PROGNOSIS

Chronic protracted course.

4.2 PANIC DISORDER

IDENTIFICATION

- Females are two to three times as likely to be affected than males, age 25–44 years, marital status, employment
- Bimodal distribution with one peak in late adolescence and a smaller peak in the mid-30s

ISSUES

Life events, life style, comorbidity, depression, suicidal ideation, drugs and alcohol.

DIFFICULTIES

Anxiety, multiple symptoms.

REFERRAL

Self, incidental, drugs and alcohol, liaison.

HISTORY OF PRESENTING COMPLAINT

Use mnemonic *FEDSA* for agoraphobia

Fear of place or situation
Escape
Difficult
Symptoms develop
Avoidance

Use mnemonic *DPIF* for panic attack

Discrete
Periods
of **I**ntense
Fear

Use mnemonic *CATASTROFIES* for panic disorder

Choking
Angina
Tachycardia
Abdominal distress
Sweat
Tremble
Rule **O**ut other anxiety disorders
Fear of dying or going crazy
Intense
Escape
SOB - short of breath

CRITERIA FOR PANIC ATTACK Modified with permission from the Diagnostic and Statistical Manual of Mental Disorders, Fourth Edition. Copyright 1994 American Psychiatric Association.

A discrete period of intense fear or discomfort in which four (or more) of the following symptoms developed abruptly and reached a peak in 10 minutes:

- Palpitations, pounding heart, or accelerated heart rate
- Sweating
- Trembling or shaking
- Sensations of shortness of breath or smothering
- Feelings of choking
- Chest pain or discomfort
- Nausea or abdominal distress
- Feeling dizzy, unsteady, light headed, or faint
- Derealization (feelings of unreality) or depersonalization (being detached from one-self)
- Fear of losing control or going crazy
- Fear of dying
- Paraesthesia (numbness or tingling sensations)
- Chills or hot flushes

DIAGNOSTIC CRITERIA FOR PANIC DISORDER WITHOUT AGORAPHOBIA Modified with permission from the Diagnostic and Statistical Manual of Mental Disorders, Fourth Edition. Copyright 1994 American Psychiatric Association.

A. Both 1 and 2.

1. Recurrent unexpected panic attacks.
2. At least one of the attacks has been followed by 1 month (or more) of one (or more) of the following:
   a. Persistent concern about having additional attacks.
   b. Worry about the implications of the attack or its consequences, e.g. losing control, having a heart attack, 'going crazy'.
   c. A significant change in behaviour related to the attacks.

B. Absence of agoraphobia.

C. The panic attacks are not due to the direct physiological effects of a substance (e.g. drug of abuse, medication) or a general medical condition (e.g. hyperthyroidism).

D. The panic attacks are not better accounted for by another mental disorder such as social phobia (e.g. occurring on exposure to feared social situations), specific phobia (e.g. on exposure to specific phobic situation), obsessive compulsive disorder (e.g. exposure to dirt in someone with an obsession about contamination), post-traumatic stress disorder (e.g. in response to stimuli associated with a severe stressor), or separation anxiety disorder (e.g. in response to being away from home or close relatives).

CRITERIA FOR AGORAPHOBIA   Modified with permission from the Diagnostic and Statistical Manual of Mental Disorders, Fourth Edition. Copyright 1994 American Psychiatric Association.

- Anxiety about being in places or situations from which escape might be difficult (or embarrassing) or in which help may not be available in the event of having an unexpected or situationally predisposed Panic attack or panic-like symptoms. Agoraphobic fears typically involve characteristic clusters of situations which include being outside the home alone, being in a crowd or standing in a line; being on a bridge; and travelling in a bus, train, automobile
- The situations are avoided (e.g. travel is restricted) or else are endured with marked distress or with anxiety about having a panic attack or panic like symptoms or require the presence of a companion
- The anxiety or phobic avoidance is not better accounted for by another mental disorder such as social phobia (e.g. avoidance limited to social situations because of fear of embarrassment), specific phobia (e.g. avoidance limited to a single situation like elevators), obsessive compulsive disorder (e.g. avoidance of dirt in someone with an obsession about contamination), posttraumatic stress disorder (e.g. avoidance of stimuli associated with a severe stressor), or separation anxiety disorder (e.g. avoidance of leaving home or relatives

Important to establish situations where fear of panic occurs and that these fearful avoidances are secondary to the basic fears – the fear of panic and its consequence (usually physical).

Onset and course

- Sudden without any obvious precipitant, may wax and wane with frequency and severity
- Associated with life events

Consequences

- Avoidance, difficulties, e.g. social, suicidality, depression, drugs and alcohol
- Average day – what do they fear/avoid? What can they do only with help?

DIFFERENTIAL DIAGNOSIS OF PANIC DISORDER

- Anxiety disorder due to a general medical condition, e.g. hyperthyroidism, hyperparathyroidism, hypoglycaemia, phaechromocytoma, vestibular dysfunctions, seizure disorders, cardiac conditions, e.g. arrthymias, supraventricular tachycardia
- Substance induced anxiety disorder, e.g. cocaine, amphetamines, caffeine, cannabis. Withdrawal from CNS depressants, e.g. alcohol, barbiturates
- Social phobia – cued by social situations
- Specific phobia – cued by object or situation
- Obsessive compulsive disorder – cued by exposure to the object of an obsession e.g. exposure to dirt in someone with an obsession about contamination
- Post-traumatic stress disorder – cued by stimuli recalling the stressor
- Separation anxiety disorder
- Delusional disorder

PANIC DISORDER: ORGANIC DIFFERENTIAL DIAGNOSIS

- Cardiovascular – anaemia, angina, congestive heart failure, hypertension, mitral valve prolapse, mitral incompetence, paroxsymal atrial tachycardia
- Pulmonary diseases – asthma, hyperventilation, pulmonary embolus
- Central nervous system – cerebrovascular disease, epilepsy, Huntington's, infection, Menieres, migraine, Multiple Sclerosis, transient ischaemic attack, tumour, Wilsons
- Endocrine – Addison's, Carcinoid, Cushing's, diabetes, hypoglycaemia, hyperthyroid, hypoparathyroid, phaechromocytoma
- Drug intoxication – amphetamines, amylnitrite, anticholinergics, cocaine, hallucinogens, marijuana, nicotine, theophylline
- Other conditions – anaphylaxis, B_{12} deficiency, porphyria, electrolyte disturbances, heavy metal poisoning, systemic infections, SLE, temporal arteritis, uraemia

Note: panic disorder can co-exist with medical conditions.

RELEVANT NEGATIVES

Depression, deliberate self harm, drugs and alcohol, cardiac disease.

FAMILY HISTORY

Psychiatric illness, anxiety, depression, drug and alcohol and suicide. Increase in family history, genetic factors.

PERSONAL HISTORY

- Early development, parenting style, separation, loss, abuse, anxiety, social, occupational, peers, inpatient relatives, support, cotherapist
- Self defeating decisions, e.g. alter job in hope that panic attacks will not recur
- Start to use drugs and alcohol to deal with situations

PAST MEDICAL HISTORY

Drug and alcohol sequelae, thyroid, diabetes, head injury, caffeine, nicotine, tobacco, substance, intoxication, withdrawal, abuse.

PAST PSYCHIATRIC HISTORY

Anxiety, depression, separation anxiety, substance dependence.

DRUG AND ALCOHOL HISTORY

Frequently dependent on substances as way of avoiding panic sensations.

PREMORBID PERSONALITY

Trait neuroticism, obsessional/perfectionist, interpersonal sensitivity, sick role, fear of future.

MENTAL STATE EXAMINATION

Impaired memory, depersonalization, derealization during an attack, anticipatory anxiety about having another attack, somatic complaints – fear of dying.

ON EXAMINATION

Increased autonomic arousal, stigmata of drugs and alcohol, thyroid.

MANAGEMENT

Safety and setting

- Clarify depressed, suicidal, drug and alcohol use, comorbidity common
- Failed outpatient

Clarify diagnosis

- Observation and disability, social interactions
- Exclude differential diagnosis

SPECIAL INVESTIGATIONS

To exclude ... I would do ...

FBC, UE, TFT, MCV, GLU, Ca, PO_4, ESR, VDRL, HIV, urinary drug screen, VMA if indicated
EEG, CT, ECG.

- Collateral history from other source to verify information
- Role of other professionals – to do what?

Establish a therapeutic alliance

Treat using a biopsychosocial model

Biological

- Role of caffeine, nicotine, stimulants
- Tricyclic antidepressants – imipramine, clomipramine
- Reduce arousal with relaxation techniques, slow breathing control for panic
- Benzodiazepines may be used in the treatment of panic disorder e.g. alprazolam

Risks of dependence and abuse. Use short-term only

- Try to educate and use slow breathing techniques to reduce reliance on benzodiazepines
- High potency benzodiazepines and tricyclics have similar efficacy to CBT packages
- These approaches may be suitable for those individuals unable to participate in a CBT programme
- Phenelzine
- Moclobemide
- Selective serotonin reuptake inhibitors – e.g. paroxetine, sertraline - slow titration of the drugs
- Treat comorbid depression, drug and alcohol withdrawal

Psychological

Establish what the primary fears are, e.g. physical harm.

Psychoeducation

- Understanding development of panic disorder, e.g. stress both psychological and physical and how to manage it, give information explaining evolution of panic attacks
- Role of hyperventilation
- Discussion of generalization of avoidance behaviours

Cognitive behavioural therapy

- Restructure false beliefs
- Hyperventilation control, teach slow breathing technique, relaxation, catastrophic interpretations and alternatives
- Graded interoceptive exposure, i.e. to panic sensations and desensitization re avoidance, homework, activity, schedule
- Relaxation and imaginal desensitization (not as effective as *in vivo*)
- Panic diary and self monitor
- Write down irrational and rational thoughts, self monitor

LONG-TERM MANAGEMENT

Safety

Decrease symptoms using a biopsychosocial approach

Chronic issues, relations, assertiveness, anxiety management.

Biological

- Treat comorbid depression with appropriate antidepressant
- Counselling for drugs and alcohol dependence

Psychological

- Cognitive behavioural therapy, relapse prevention
- Social – guard against avoidance, rehabilitation issues, life style
- Encourage social skills and family support, education and culture
- Psychodynamic psychotherapy may help identify psychosocial variables which play a part in the development of an active vulnerability to panic attacks, also if there is secondary gain in remaining 'ill' which enables the person to avoid making decisions about what else to do with his/her life

PROGNOSIS

- Life events, motivation, comorbidity, relative strengths
- Panic disorder – 30–40% patients are symptom free at long-term follow up, 50% have symptoms which are mild enough not to effect their lives significantly, 10–20% continue to have significant symptoms
- Panic disorder with agoraphobia tends to improve with treatment of the panic disorder and with cognitive behavioural therapy
- Best indicator is degree of avoidance at end of treatment – note: beware subtle avoidance.
- Agoraphobia without a history of panic disorder is often chronic. There are often comorbid disorders of depression and alcohol dependence

4.3 SOCIAL PHOBIA

IDENTIFICATION

- Female almost equal sex ratio (1.2:1), greater than male, age 25–44 years, marital status, employment
- Prevalence 3–13%

ISSUES

Life events, life style, comorbidity, depression, suicidal ideation, drugs and alcohol.

DIFFICULTIES

Anxiety, avoidance of situations, restricted lifestyle.

REFERRAL

Self, drugs and alcohol, liaison.

HISTORY OF PRESENTING COMPLAINT

- Experiences panic attacks in certain situations
- Symptoms; especially blushing, sweating and shaking

DIAGNOSTIC CRITERIA FOR SOCIAL PHOBIA Modified with permission from the Diagnostic and Statistical Manual of Mental Disorders, Fourth Edition. Copyright 1994 American Psychiatric Association.

- A marked and persistent fear of one or more social or performance situations in which the person is exposed to unfamiliar people or to possible scrutiny by others. The individual fears that he or she will act in a way (or show anxiety symptoms) that will be humiliating or embarrassing
- Exposure to the feared social situation almost invariably provokes anxiety, which may take the form of a situationally bound or situationally predisposed panic attack
- The person recognises that the fear is excessive or unreasonable
- The feared social or performance situations are avoided or else are endured with intense anxiety or distress

- The avoidance, anxious anticipation or distress in the feared social or performance situation(s) interferes significantly with the persons normal routine, occupational (academic) functioning or social activities or relationships or there is marked distress about having the phobia
- In individuals under age 18 years the duration is at least 6 months
- The fear or avoidance is not due to the direct physiological effects of a substance (e.g. a drug of abuse, a medication) or a general medical condition and is not better accounted for by another mental disorder (e.g. panic disorder with or without agoraphobia, separation anxiety disorder, body dysmorphic disorder, a pervasive developmental disorder or schizoid personality disorder)
- If a general medical condition or another mental disorder is present the fear in the first criteria unrelated to it, e.g. the fear is not of stuttering, trembling in Parkinson's disease or exhibiting abnormal eating behaviour in anorexia nervosa or bulimia nervosa

Specify if generalized – if the fears include most social situations (also consider the additional diagnosis of avoidant personality disorder)

Common situations:

- Speaking on the phone
- Writing in front of others
- Entering a room
- Parties
- Public speaking
- Using public toilet
- Eating or drinking in public
- Public transport
- Queues
- Crowds

Note: very similar to agoraphobia but distinguished by cognitions (agoraphobia – fear of inability to escape or help being unavailable).

Cognitions

- Fears being the centre of attention
- Fear of scrutiny
- Fear of embarrassment
- Fear of appearing foolish
- Fear of negative evaluation

Onset and course

In the mid-teens, sometimes emerging from a childhood history of social inhibition or shyness. Course is continuous and the duration life long, although it may wax and wane in severity. Stressors have impact on impairment.

Consequences

- Avoidance, e.g. social, suicidality, depression, drugs and alcohol
- Average day, restricted life style
- Seeking help now due to restrictions it has imposed on life

DIFFERENTIAL DIAGNOSIS

- Panic disorder with agoraphobia
- Agoraphobia without a history of panic disorder
- Separation anxiety disorder
- Generalized anxiety disorder
- Specific phobia
- Pervasive developmental disorder
- Schizoid personality disorder
- Avoidant personality disorder
- Associated features of many other mental disorders, e.g. major depressive disorder, dysthymic disorder, Schizophrenia, body dysmorphic disorder
- Anxiety disorder not otherwise specified
- Performance Anxiety, stage fright, shyness
- Anxiety disorder due to a general medical condition, e.g. hyperthyroidism, hyperparathyroidism, hypoglycaemia, phaechromocytoma, vestibular dysfunctions, seizure disorders, cardiac conditions, e.g. arrhythmias, supraventricular tachycardia

PANIC DISORDER: ORGANIC DIFFERENTIAL DIAGNOSIS

- Cardiovascular – anaemia, angina, congestive heart failure, hypertension, mitral valve prolapse, mitral incompetence, paroxsymal atrial tachycardia
- Pulmonary diseases – asthma, hyperventilation, pulmonary embolus
- Central nervous system – cerebrovascular disease, epilepsy, Huntington's, infection, Menieres, migraine, Multiple Sclerosis, transient ischaemic attack, tumour, Wilsons
- Endocrine – Addison's, carcinoid, Cushing's, diabetes, hypoglycaemia, hyperthyroid, hypoparathyroid, phaechromocytoma
- Drug intoxication – amphetamines, amylnitrite, anticholinergics, cocaine, hallucinogens, marijuana, nicotine, theophylline
- Other conditions – anaphalaxis, B_{12} deficiency, porphyria, electrolyte disturbances, heavy metal poisoning, systemic infections, SLE, temporal arteritis, uraemia

RELEVANT NEGATIVES

Depression, deliberate self harm, drugs and alcohol, cardiac disease.

FAMILY HISTORY

Psychiatric illness, anxiety, depression, drug and alcohol and suicide. Increase in family history in first degree biological relatives.

PERSONAL HISTORY

Early development, parenting style including interactional style, separation, loss, abuse, anxiety, social, occupational, peers, relatives, previous relationships, friendships, type of friends and support.

PAST MEDICAL HISTORY

Drug and alcohol sequelae, thyroid, diabetes, head injury, caffeine, nicotine, tobacco, substance intoxication, withdrawal, abuse.

PAST PSYCHIATRIC HISTORY

Anxiety, depression, separation anxiety.

PREMORBID PERSONALITY

- Trait neuroticism, obsessional/perfectionist, interpersonal sensitivity, sick role, fear of future
- Cluster C traits usually, sometimes Cluster B

MENTAL STATE EXAMINATION

- Decreased eye contact, ill at ease, speech hesitant
- Impaired memory, depersonalization, derealization during an attack, anticipatory anxiety about having another attack

ON EXAMINATION

Increased autonomic arousal, stigmata of drugs and alcohol, thyroid.

MANAGEMENT

Safety and setting

- Clarify if depressed, suicidal, drug and alcohol use, comorbidity common
- Failed outpatient

Clarify diagnosis

- Observation and disability, social interactions
- Exclude differential diagnosis

SPECIAL INVESTIGATIONS

To exclude ... I would do ...

FBC, UE, TFT, MCV, GLU, Ca, PO_4. ESR. VDRL. HIV. urinary drug screen. VMA. if indicated EEG. CT. ECG.

Fear of Negative Evaluation Scale.

Social Avoidance and Distress Scale.

Often comorbid personality disorder especially Cluster C, avoidant personality disorder.

Comorbidity estimates of avoidant personality disorder with social phobia vary from 22 to 84%.

May use Personality Disorder Examination (Loranger 1988) to gain more information.

Comorbidity with other axis I disorders is high, e.g. other anxiety disorders, depression, substance dependence especially alcohol which is commonly used as an anxiolytic.

- Collateral history from other source to verify information
- Role of other professionals – to do what?

Establish a therapeutic alliance

Treat using a biopsychosocial model

Biological

Role of caffeine, nicotine, stimulants – avoid.

β blockers, e.g. propranolol may reduce peripheral symptoms resulting from hyperactivity of the adrenergic system, e.g. tremor, sweating, blushing, dry mouth, palpitations. They are often used to help performance anxiety. Beware a history of asthma. Does not help change underlying cognitions of the disorder.

Benzodiazepines. Helps reduce symptoms of anxiety, risk of relapse when medication withdrawn, risk of dependency, does not deal with underlying cognitions

Monoamine oxidase inhibitors

- Phenelzine, moclobemide – high doses
- Improvement of symptoms in social phobia and social phobia with avoidant personality disorder
- Relapse is common after discontinuation

Selective serotonin reuptake inhibitors. Treat comorbid depression

Treat drug and alcohol withdrawal.

Psychological

1. Psychoeducation
2. Cognitive Behavioural Therapy

- Preferably a group treatment (exposes the individual to others with the condition so they become aware that 'not just me') rather than individual treatment. Acts as exposure task as have to be with and interact with others
- Education re: nature of social phobia and panic attacks and physiology
- Hyperventilation control, slow breathing techniques, relaxation
- Restructure false beliefs, irrational, unhelpful thoughts, catastrophic interpretations and alternatives, likelihood and consequences of negative evaluation
- Graded exposure and desensitization, avoidance, homework, activity
- Imaginal desensitization
- Diary and self monitor thoughts and tasks
- Structured problem solving
- Assertiveness
- Setbacks and continued treatment strategies

LONG-TERM MANAGEMENT

Safety

Decrease symptoms using a biopsychosocial approach

Chronic issues, relations, assertiveness, anxiety management.

Biological

Antidepressant if indicated, comorbid depression and drugs and alcohol.

Psychological

- Cognitive behavioural therapy has long-term benefits, relapse prevention, guard against avoidance, rehabilitation issues, life style
- Social skills and family support, education and culture

PROGNOSIS

- Chronic illness with average onset in mid–late teens
- Life events, motivation, comorbidity, relative strengths
- The long term outcome is related to the cognitive component of the treatment and success of the cognitive restructuring
- Outcome is also related to the severity of the initial symptoms

SHYNESS

- Shyness may result in some mild social anxiety that involves some fear of negative evaluation but does not lead to significant distress or avoidance. Prevalence rate 40%
- Social anxiety develops in adolescence

AVOIDANT PERSONALITY DISORDER

- Commonly comorbid
- Controversy re: ?separation disorder
- Display a fear of rejection and sense of inferiority
- Poor response to treatment

4.4 OBSESSIVE COMPULSIVE DISORDER

IDENTIFICATION

- Male = female, lifetime prevalence of 2.5%
- Age, sex, marital status, living with, employment, culture

REFERRAL

Self, school, family.

ISSUES

Onset in adolescence or early 20s (developmental), impairment in functioning, comorbidity, depression, chronicity.

DIFFICULTIES

Embarrassment, guarded.

HISTORY OF PRESENTING COMPLAINT

Use mnemonic *RESIDENT PRISONER*

Recurrent ideas
Experienced as
Senseless and attempt to
Ignore ideas
Drugs – rule out
Eating disorder – rule out
Not related to
Thought insertion – rule out

Purposeful
Repetitive
Intentional
Stereotyped

response to **O**bsession
Neutralization
Excessive
interfere with **R**outine

DIAGNOSTIC CRITERIA FOR OBSESSIVE COMPULSIVE DISORDER   Modified with permission from the Diagnostic and Statistical Manual of Mental Disorders, Fourth Edition. Copyright 1994 American Psychiatric Association.

A. Either obsessions or compulsions. Obsessions as defined by 1–4

1. Recurrent and persistent thoughts, impulses, or images that are experienced, at some time during the disturbance, as intrusive and inappropriate and that cause marked anxiety or distress.
2. The thoughts, impulses or images are not simply excessive worries about real-life problems.
3. The person attempts to ignore or suppress such thoughts, impulses or images, or to neutralize them with some other thought or action.
4. The person recognizes that the obsessional thoughts impulses or images are a product of his or her own mind (not imposed from without as in thought insertion).

Compulsions as defined by (1) and (2)

(1) Repetitive behaviours (e.g. hand washing, ordering, checking or mental acts, e.g. praying, counting, repeating words silently) that the person feels driven to perform in response to an obsession, or according to rules that must be applied rigidly.
(2) The behaviours or mental acts are aimed at preventing or reducing distress or preventing some dreaded event or situation; however these behaviours or mental acts either are not connected in a realistic way with what they are designed to neutralize or prevent or are clearly excessive.

B. At some point during the course of the disorder, the person has recognized that the obsessions or compulsions are excessive or unreasonable (note this does not apply to children).

C. The obsessions or compulsions cause marked distress, are time consuming (take more than one hour a day) or significantly interfere with the persons normal routine, occupational (or academic) functioning or usual social activities or relationships.

D. If another axis 1 disorder is present the content of the obsessions or compulsion is not restricted to it

E. The disturbance is not due to the direct physiological effects of a substance (e.g. a drug of abuse, a medication) or a general medical condition.

Specify: **with poor insight:** if for most of the time during the current episode, the person does not recognize that the obsessions and compulsions are excessive or unreasonable.

Obsession ⟶ fear of harm ⟶ compulsion ⟶ neutralize risk

OBSESSION

A recurrent intrusive thought, feeling, idea or sensation which is perceived as unreasonable.

- Obsessional thoughts, impulses, images, contamination, doubt, obsessional slowness. Presence of compulsions and resistance and whether any situations avoided because of it. Guilt
- Commonest are contamination, intrusive thoughts without a compulsion (violence, sex and blasphemy), sameness, lucky and unlucky numbers, doubt

COMPULSION

A conscious, standardized (ritual) recurrent thought or behaviour, e.g. counting, checking or avoiding which occurs in response to the obsession

- Compulsions, e.g. hand wash and grooming, rituals, checking, touching (aim: prevent harm to self and loved ones), counting, hoarding and collecting
- Adolesence, adulthood, precipitant and course
- Age of onset is earlier in men 6–15 years and 20–29 years for women. Onset gradual, wax and wane and exacerbation of symptoms are related to stress
- Aim of compulsions is to minimize or eliminate risk of feared consequence
- Rituals have no accompanying resistance and are usually based on some magical or superstitious belief i.e. throwing spilt salt over shoulder

RELEVANT NEGATIVES

Psychotic, bizarre, egosyntonic, depression, anxiety disorder, especially generalized anxiety disorder with its worries and obsessions, suicidality, drugs and alcohol, eating disorder.

CONSEQUENCES

- For relations, family, peers, school, occupation, activities
- Severity – impairment in functioning, time involved, disruption to other members of household

FAMILY HISTORY

- Concordance rate is higher for monozygotic twins, increase risk in first degree relatives of obsessive compulsive disorder 21–25 % and those with Tourettes disorder, approximately 17% obsessive compulsive traits and 5% have multiple tics
- Increased risk of obsessive compulsive disorder, Gilles de la Tourette Syndrome, anxiety, affective disorders, suicide, drugs and alcohol

PERSONAL HISTORY

- Birth, development, early childhood, separation, loss, abuse, school, occupation, psychosexual, peers and interests. Current level of functioning – social, life events, occupation, interpersonal relativity, family attitudes (limited relevance to aetiology)
- 15 % have symptoms before age of 10 years. Females report an increase in symptoms around the time of their periods. Age of onset is earlier in males than in females. Frequent marital problems

PAST MEDICAL HISTORY

Prenatal trauma, head injury, epilepsy, temporal lobe epilepsy, effective treatment and progress, iatrogenic.

PAST PSYCHIATRIC HISTORY

Depression, anxiety disorder, separation anxiety, tic disorder, suicidal ideation, deliberate self harm, autism, Asperger, can be a precursor to schizophrenia.

DRUGS AND ALCOHOL

Past and present use of benzodiazepines, self medication.

PREMORBID PERSONALITY

- Cluster C – avoidant, dependent, obsessive-compulsive
- Cluster A – schizoid
- Coping mechanisms, proneness to anxiety and strengths
- Psychodynamic theory – isolation, undoing, reaction formation and displacement

MENTAL STATE EXAMINATION

- Behaviour, affect, mood, thought form, content, obsessions and compulsions, exclude psychotic symptoms, insight, cognition
- Insight – recognize the irrationality of experiences and that they are ego dystonic

ON EXAMINATION

- Pulse and Blood Pressure – over aroused
- Signs of dermatological problems
- Closely observe behaviour – touching, not touching, checking

MANAGEMENT

Safety

- Treat comorbid depression, symptoms and rehabilitate
- Inpatient treatment only if severely depressed or failed outpatient
- Assessment instruments e.g. Yale–Brown Obsessive Compulsive Scale
- or Maudsley Obsessive Compulsive Scale

Clarify primary diagnosis

- Observations and disability – type of behaviour
- Exclude differential diagnosis

Ego syntonic or pleasurable thoughts are not OCD, i.e. exhibitionism is not a compulsion.

DIFFERENTIAL DIAGNOSIS

Anxiety disorder due to a general medical condition

- Endocrine, e.g. hyper and hypothyroidism, phaechromocytoma, hypoglycaemia, hyperadrenocorticism)
- Cardiovascular conditions, e.g. congestive heart failure, pulmonary embolus, arrhythmia
- Respiratory – chronic obstructive pulmonary disease, pulmonary disease, pneumonia, hyperventilation
- Metabolic conditions – e.g. vitamin B_{12} deficiency, porphyria
- Neurological conditions – neoplasms, vestibular dysfunction, encephalitis

Other possible causes

- Substance induced anxiety disorder e.g. drugs of abuse, medication. exposure to a toxin
- Body dysmorphic disorder
- Specific or social phobia
- Trichotillomania
- Major depressive episode – 30% of patients have obsessive compulsive character traits, e.g. guilt
- Generalized anxiety disorder
- Hypochondriasis
- Specific phobia
- Delusional disorder or psychotic disorder not otherwise specified
- Schizophrenia – magical thinking
- Tic disorder – 30–50% of Gilles de la Tourette patients have OCD. Touching rituals are more common
- Eating disorders
- Paraphilias
- Pathological gambling
- Alcohol dependence or abuse
- Obsessive-compulsive personality disorder
- Superstitions and repetitive checking behaviours

COMORBIDITY

Depression and other anxiety disorders and cluster C, obsessive-compulsive personality disorder, GTS.

- Collateral history from school, partner, referring agent
- Role of other professionals – to do what?

Establish therapeutic alliance

Decrease symptoms using a biopsychosocial model

Often best results achieved with joint biological and CBT programme

Biological

Exposure and response prevention
- If necessary use adjunct drug treatment
- SSRI are effective, e.g. fluoxetine 20-80 mg/day, paroxetine 40-60 mg/day, fluvoxamine 100-300 mg, sertraline 50-200mg
- Clomipramine up to 250 mg daily in divided doses. Start at 25–50 mg at night and increase by 25 mg every 2–3 days. Side effects : hypotension, sedation, sexual dysfunction and anticholinergic side effects
- Length of treatment – some patients respond only after 8 weeks of treatment although often not until 8–16 weeks to get maximum therapeutic effect. Continue medication for 1 year
- NB relapse is usual
- Treat comorbid disorders

Psychological

- Cognitive behaviour therapy
- Psychoeducation re nature and symptoms of OCD
- *In vivo* exposure and response prevention – deliberate exposure to avoided situations, direct exposure to feared stimulus, prevention of compulsive rituals and neutralizing behaviours
- Participant modelling – initial stages
- Design programme to cues and triggers
- Start exposure tasks

- Desensitization – anxiety reduction procedures are based on the principle that resisting the compulsive behaviours/urges will reduce or eliminate the anxiety associated with obsessions. This will eventually extinguish the compulsive behaviours
- Rehearsal and imagery in session
- Use daily home work and assignments, practise
- Commitment of patient paramount

LONG-TERM MANAGEMENT

- Relationship with patient, compliance and side effects of medication
- Psychosurgery – cingulotomy, anterior capsulotomy or modified leucotomy in severe intractable OCD which has not responded to traditional treatments
- Stereotactic safe, complications are post operative seizures in 1% of patients

AETIOLOGY

Theories

- Link with character trait
- The superego defences are used as the psychic apparatus has regressed to the preoedipal, anal and sadistic phase
- Isolation is a defence mechanism that protects a person from anxiety provoking effects and impulses
- Undoing – the compulsive act will reduce anxiety
- Reaction formation – manifest in attitudes that are the opposite of underlying impulses.
- Ambivalence – love and hate towards an object therefore doing and undoing
- Magical thinking – regression uncovers early modes of thought. People think they can bring about an external event by thinking about it
- Biological studies show that PET has elevated metabolic rates in the cingulate region and the heads of the caudate nuclei and orbital gyri and frontal lobes
- Content of the obsessions, e.g. sexual/violent are thoughts in all human beings, e.g. in unconscious processes such as dreams. These are normally suppressed by striatal mechanisms during development. A dysfunctional striatum allows the intrusion of these adventitious thoughts and sensations into conscious awareness while the mental process is otherwise engaged
- Serotonin subsystem dysfunction – prefrontal cortex and striatum are rich in serotonin, the chief neurotransmitter implicated in OCD. OCD is helped by serotonin blocking drugs

PROGNOSIS

- It is a relapsing condition
- 75% improve with cognitive behavioural therapy, possibility of long-term maintenance gains

- 20–30 % significant improvement, 40–50 % have moderate improvement
- 20–40% of patients remain ill
- Obsessions without compulsions have a worse prognosis if depressed
- Suicide is a risk
- Anticipate difficulties, anxiety reduction, failure to progress, non compliance, failure to generalize

4.5 POST-TRAUMATIC STRESS DISORDER

IDENTIFICATION

Age, sex, ex-service, war veteran, culture, refugee, occupation, marital status, cohabit.

ISSUES

Chronicity, disability, comorbidity, cultural issues in management.

REFERRED

Spouse, organisation, drug and alcohol services, self.

HISTORY OF PRESENTING COMPLAINT

Need to know personal meaning of the trauma – safety violations and subsequent impact of the dysfunction.

Use mnemonic *DREAMS*

Disinterest and detachment
Re-experience nightmares and flashbacks
Events, type or single trauma, multiple
Avoidance of the situations, thoughts that invoke trauma
Month – greater than one
Sympathetic hyperactivity, exaggerated startle response

DIAGNOSTIC CRITERIA FOR POST-TRAUMATIC STRESS DISORDER Modified with permission from the Diagnostic and Statistical Manual of Mental Disorders, Fourth Edition. Copyright 1994 American Psychiatric Association.

A. The person has been exposed to a traumatic event in which both of the following were present:

- The person experienced, witnessed, or was confronted with an event or events that involved actual or threatened death or serious injury or a threat to the physical integrity of self or others
- The persons response involved intense fear, helplessness or horror

B. The traumatic event is re experienced in one (or more) of the following ways:

- Recurrent and intrusive distressing recollections of the event including images, thoughts or perceptions
- Recurrent distressing dreams of the event
- Acting or feeling as if the traumatic event were recurring (includes a sense of reliving the experience, illusions, hallucinations, and dissociative flashback episodes, including those that occur on awakening or when intoxicated)
- Intense psychological distress at exposure to internal or external cues that symbolise or resemble an aspect of the traumatic event
- Physiological reactivity on exposure to internal or external cues that symbolise or resemble an aspect of the traumatic event

C. Persistent avoidance of stimuli associated with the trauma and numbing of general responsiveness as indicated by three (or more) of the following:

- Efforts to avoid thoughts, feelings, or conversations associated with the trauma
- Efforts to avoid activities, places or people that arouse recollections of the trauma
- Inability to recall an important aspect of the trauma
- Markedly diminished interest or participation in significant activities
- Feeling of detachment or estrangement from others
- Restricted range of affect (e.g. unable to have loving feelings)
- Sense of a foreshortened future (does not expect to have career, marriage, children, or a normal life span)

D. Persistent symptoms of increased arousal (not present before the trauma) as indicated by two (or more) of the following:

- Difficulty in staying asleep or falling asleep
- Irritability or outbursts of anger
- Difficulty in concentrating
- Hypervigilance
- Exaggerated startle response

E. Duration of the disturbance (symptoms in criteria B–D) is >1 month.

F. The disturbance causes clinically significant distress or impairment in social, occupational or other important areas of functioning.

Specify if:

- Acute: duration of symptoms <3 months
- Chronic: duration of symptoms 3 months or more
- With delayed onset: if onset of symptoms is at least 6 months after the stressor

- Onset – immediate, long latency, episodic, past exacerbations

RELEVANT NEGATIVES

Deliberate self harm, drugs and alcohol, depression.

CONSEQUENCES

Problems with occupation, relationships, forensic disabilities, handicap, anxiety, depression, drugs and alcohol, suicide.

PERSONAL HISTORY

Childhood trauma. Level of functioning pretrauma and discrepancy from past level. Social relationships and occupation.

PAST MEDICAL HISTORY

Physical effects, alcohol, injuries, torture, physical disabilities.

PAST PSYCHIATRIC HISTORY

Pre-existing pathology, depression, anxiety, post-traumatic stress disorder, drugs and alcohol.

PREMORBID PERSONALITY

- Pre event level of neuroticism and post event difficulty expressing emotion and not getting involved
- Forensic impulsivity and acting out violence
- Social isolation as estranged from family and friends

MENTAL STATE EXAMINATION

Restricted display of emotion and difficulty in rapport, cognitions about event and refusal to comment, alexithymic.

ON EXAMINATION

Sequelae of trauma or substance abuse.

MANAGEMENT

Safety and setting

Containment if suicidal or depressed

May need to detox (comorbid diagnosis)

Clarify diagnosis

- Observations and disability
- Exclude differential diagnosis

DIFFERENTIAL DIAGNOSIS

- Adjustment disorder
- Acute stress disorder
- Obsessive compulsive disorder
- Schizophrenia
- Mood disorder with psychotic features
- Delirium
- Substance induced disorders
- Psychotic disorders due to a general medical condition
- Malingering
- Anxiety Disorders
- Personality disorders

PTSD shares characteristic symptoms with depression, anxiety and dissociative disorders often causing misdiagnosis

Treat comorbidity which is common e.g. affective, anxiety disorders and substance dependence

SPECIAL INVESTIGATIONS

To exclude ... I would do ...

Justify necessity for tests

EMG, Heart rate, sweat gland activity show increased autonomic arousal.

- Collateral history from other sources to verify information, history, old notes, discharge summaries, inpatient evidence
- Role of other professionals – to do what?

Establish a therapeutic alliance

Decrease symptoms using a biopsychosocial model

Biological

- Antidepressant if indicated at therapeutic doses
- Benzodiazepines often used for short term management

Psychosocial

- Education re psychological responses to traumatic stress
- Type of trauma and cultural differences important
- Goal to restore emotional control and pre trauma level of behaviour
- Counter transference issues
- Rapport and alliance and catharsis in a safe environment, here and now advocacy
- Education support, cognitive behavioural therapy
- Education about diagnosis and counter stigma
- Monitor dysfunctional thoughts and behaviour
- Teach coping skills, e.g. problem solving, assertion, relaxation
- Graded exposure to past enjoyable functional activities
- Dynamic reconstruction of the trauma may be helpful

LONG-TERM MANAGEMENT

Psychosocial

- Monitor symptoms and functioning level, comorbid pathology may require treatment, encourage skills maintenance, coping skills, assertiveness, relaxation, encourage purposeful and positive activity and ongoing support
- Dynamic – with time and rapport may deal with defences, i.e. denial, repression, defensive numbing and reaction formation, spouse/partner issues, self help group

Litigation issues

- Often a major part of treatment, symptoms may not resolve until after legal process finished

Good prognosis

Associated with:

- Rapid onset
- Short duration
- Good premorbid functioning
- Social support
- Lack of comorbid substance abuse
- Lack of psychiatric diagnoses

Vulnerability to PTSD:

- Childhood trauma
- Other psychiatric disorders
- Inadequate support
- Genetic predisposition to psychiatric vulnerability
- Stressful life changes
- External locus of control
- Increased alcohol intake

Look for secondary gain – compensation, attention, etc.

SUBSTANCE-RELATED DISORDERS

5.1 ALCOHOL

REFERRAL

Accident and Emergency, outpatients, self, family, police.

IDENTIFICATION

- Age, culture, occupation, marital status
- Male onset in teens and 20s
- Clinical index of suspicion due to early symptoms and signs of alcohol dependence, intoxication, alcohol-related disease, history of excessive intake
- Common

HISTORY PRESENTING COMPLAINT

- Thorough drinking and alcohol history, onset, early experience, course, when, where, with whom, salience, clinical presentation, last 3 drinking occasions, amount, pattern of use, symptoms, e.g. blackouts, tremors, withdrawal seizures, withdrawal delirium, cerebrovascular accounts, medical sequelae, laboratory markers MCV and GGT, use of other drugs
- Corroborative history
- Features of dependence listed below:

CRITERIA FOR SUBSTANCE ABUSE   Modified with permission from the Diagnostic and Statistical Manual of Mental Disorders, Fourth Edition. Copyright 1994 American Psychiatric Association.

A maladaptive pattern of substance use, leading to clinically significant impairment or distress as manifested by three (or more) of the following, occurring at any time during the same 12-month period:

A. Tolerance, as defined by either:

- A need for markedly increased amounts of the substance to achieve intoxication or desired effect.
- Markedly diminished effect with continued use of the same amount of the substance.

B. Withdrawal, as manifested by either:

- The characteristic withdrawal syndrome for the substance
- The same (or closely related) substance is taken to relieve or avoid withdrawal symptoms

C. The substance is often taken in larger amounts or over a longer period than was intended.

D. There is a persistent desire or unsuccessful efforts to cut down or control substance use.

E. A great deal of time is spent in activities necessary to obtain the substance (e.g. visiting doctors or driving long distances), use the substance (e.g. chain smoking), or recover from its effects.

E. Important social or occupational or recreational activities are given up or reduced because of substance use.

F. The substance use is continued despite knowledge of having a persistent or recurrent physical or psychological problem that is likely to have been caused or exacerbated by the substance.

Specify if:

- With Physiological dependence: evidence of tolerance or withdrawal
- Without Physiological dependence: no evidence of tolerance or withdrawal

Course specifiers:

- Early full remission – for at least 1 month but for <12 months no criteria for dependence or abuse were met
- Early partial remission – >1 month but <12 months one or more of the criteria for dependence or abuse were met
- Sustained full remission – none of the criteria for Dependence or abuse have been met at any time during 12 months
- Sustained partial remission - criteria for Dependence not met for 12 months or longer but one or more criteria for Dependence/Abuse have been met
- On Agonist Therapy - on agonist medication, no criteria for Dependence or Abuse met for at least 1 month (except tolerance or withdrawal from agonist)
- In a Controlled Environment - environment where access to alcohol and controlled substances is restricted and no criteria for Dependence or Abuse have been met for at least the past month

CRITERIA FOR SUBSTANCE ABUSE Modified with permission from the Diagnostic and Statistical Manual of Mental Disorders, Fourth Edition. Copyright 1994 American Psychiatric Association.

A maladaptive pattern of substance use leading to clinically significant impairment or distress as manifested by one (or more) of the following occuring within a 12-month period:

- Recurrent substance use resulting in a failure to fulfil major role obligations at work, school, home (e.g. repeated absences or poor work-related performance related to substance use; substance-related absences, suspensions or expulsions from school; neglect of children or household)
- Recurrent substance use in situations in which it is physically hazardous (e.g. driving an automobile, or operating a machine when impaired by substance use)
- Recurrent substance-related legal problems (e.g. arrests for substance-related disorderly conduct)

- Continued substance use despite having persistent or recurrent social or interpersonal problems caused or exacerbated by the effects of the substance (e.g. arguments with spouse about the consequences of intoxication, physical fights)

The symptoms have never met the criteria for substance dependence for this class of substance.

DIAGNOSTIC CRITERIA FOR ALCOHOL INTOXICATION   Modified with permission from the Diagnostic and Statistical Manual of Mental Disorders, Fourth Edition. Copyright 1994 American Psychiatric Association.

A. Recent ingestion of alcohol

B. Clinically significant maladaptive behavioural or psychological changes (e.g. inappropriate sexual or aggressive behaviour, mood lability, impaired judgement, impaired social or occupational functioning) that developed during or shortly after alcohol ingestion.

C. One (or more) of the following signs develop during or shortly after alcohol use:

- Slurred speech
- Incoordination
- Unsteady gait
- Nystagmus
- Impairment in attention or memory
- Stupor or coma

The symptoms are not accounted for by a general medical condition and are not better accounted for by another mental disorder.

DIFFERENTIAL DIAGNOSIS

- Head trauma
- Hepatic encephalopathy
- Infection, e.g. meningitis or encephalitis
- Post-ictal states
- Intoxication caused by sedative hypnotic drugs
- Severe hypoglycaemia

TREATMENT

Supportive

- Thiamine 100 mg intramuscularly then orally
- Multivitamin preparation including B vitamins and folate
- Benzodiazepine or antipychotic, e.g. haloperidol to calm the patient
- Comatose intoxicated patient – thiamine 100 mg intravenously to protect against Wernicke's and glucose intravenously to correct for alcohol induced hypoglycaemia
- 5% of individuals with alcohol dependence will have complications of withdrawal
- However elective withdrawal is usually uncomplicated if the person is in good health

DIAGNOSTIC CRITERIA FOR ALCOHOL WITHDRAWAL Modified with permission from the Diagnostic and Statistical Manual of Mental Disorders, Fourth Edition. Copyright 1994 American Psychiatric Association.

A. Cessation of (or reduction in) alcohol use that has been heavy and prolonged.

B. Two (or more) of the following, developing within several hours to a few days after Criterion A:

- Autonomic hyperactivity, e.g. sweat, pulse rate >100 beats per min
- Increased hand tremor
- Insomnia
- Nausea or vomiting
- Transient visual, auditory, tactile hallucinations or illusions
- Psychomotor agitation
- Anxiety
- Grand mal seizures

C. The symptoms above cause clinically significant distress or impairment in social, occupational, or other important areas of functioning.

D. The symptoms are not due to a general medical condition and are not better accounted for by another medical disorder.

Specify if:

With perceptual disturbances

Seizures

Occur 7–48 hours after cessation. One-third of patients will only have one seizure and two-thirds have closely spaced outbursts of seizures. 2% have status epilepticus and underlying seizure disorder.

Check

Check other causes for seizures, e.g. head injury, central nervous system infection, neoplasm, cerebrovascular disease, hypoglycaemia, hyponatraemia, hypomagnesaemia.

Early mild symptoms of withdrawal

Autonomic over activity (tachycardia, hypertension, fever, tremor, restless, irritable and hostility, agitation, startle response), distractible or poor concentration, anorexia, nausea and vomiting, diarrhoea, weak, cramps, insomnia, nightmares.

Major symptoms of withdrawal

Visual, auditory, tactile hallucinations, delusions, disorientation to time and place (part of clouding of consciousness), fluctuating course and worsening of symptoms and signs of early syndrome, seizures.

TREATMENT OF WITHDRAWAL

- Good nursing care
- Tranquil, well-lit space and familiar visitors
- Abstinence from alcohol
- Rest, nutrition
- Reality orientation, day, date, surroundings
- Loading dose of 20 mg diazepam 2 hours until sedated or a maximum of 100 mg/day as titrate dose to symptoms
- Hydration – give oral fluids and food
- Vitamins – thiamine 100 mg intramuscularly then orally
- Oral multivitamins
- Haloperidol for hallucinations, give concomitantly with benzodiazepines, not alone

Delirium Tremens

This is an uncommon manifestation. Appears after 1–4 days. Mortality is high, 15% in the presence of medical illness (pneumonia, renal disease and hepatic insufficiency or heart failure). Develops in patients after 5–15 years of heavy drinking of the binge type.

- Reduce environmental stimuli
- Use a well-lit room and explain all the procedures
- Monitor electrolytes and fluid balance
- Give thiamine 100 mg intramuscularly then 100 mg tds orally and folate, B complex and multivitamin supplements. Thiamine is given prior to a glucose load or thiamine levels are depleted and could precipitate Wernickes
- Give chlormethiazole four capsules qds and then titrate against symptoms
- Haloperidol needed if paranoid or hallucinations
- High calorie and high carbohydrate diet
- Treat any complicating illnesses

DIFFERENTIAL DIAGNOSIS OF ALCOHOL-INDUCED DISORDERS

- Primary mental disorders, e.g. depression, anxiety
- General medical conditions, e.g. diabetic acidosis, cerebellar ataxia, multiple sclerosis, hypoglycaemia, diabetic ketoacidosis
- Essential tremor
- Sedative, hypnotic, anxiolytic intoxication/withdrawal
- Alcohol induced disorders
- Alcohol idiosyncratic intoxication – alcohol-related disorder not otherwise specified

FAMILY HISTORY

Genetic component

Strong family history and coexistence of substance abuse.

PERSONAL HISTORY

- Early environment, conduct disorder, occupation, e.g. journalists, publicans, hospitality industry
- Current financial difficulty – frequently in debt due to job loss

PAST MEDICAL HISTORY

Sequelae of alcohol abuse:

- Central nervous system – head injury, epilepsy, ataxia, neuropathy, memory deficit, alcohol related brain damage
- Gastrointestinal tract – liver, bleeds, melaena, pain, pancreatitis
- Respiratory tract – increased infection, e.g. tuberculosis, increased risk if smoking
- HIV, hepatitis B and C
- Attention deficit hyperactivity disorder

PAST PSYCHIATRIC HISTORY

- Comorbidity is common in the majority of patients, e.g. antisocial personality disorder, phobias, depressive disorder, opioid dependence and dysthymia
- 15% of those with alcohol abuse or dependence commit suicide
- Deliberate self harm is common
- Alcohol problem may present as anxiety disorder or morbid jealousy

DRUGS

Use of illicit drugs.

PREMORBID PERSONALITY

Low self esteem.

MENTAL STATE EXAMINATION

Anxiety, depression, perceptions, delusional jealousy, frontal lobe signs.

ON EXAMINATION

- Intoxication, withdrawal symptoms
- Central nervous system – Wernickes, opthalmoplegia, ataxia, nystagmus, confusion, alcohol-related brain damage
- Chronic sequelae – GIT, central nervous system

- Respiratory system – intercurrent infection
- Nutritional state
- Signs of other drug use, tattoos – artistic or institutional

MANAGEMENT

Safety and dangerousness

Comorbid diagnosis?

Patients intoxicated or in delirium due to withdrawal may be at risk to themselves and others.

Clarify diagnosis

- Observations and disability
- Collaborative history, old notes, relations, friends, nursing observations, interactions with staff or on the ward
- Exclude differential diagnosis e.g. infection, subdural haemotoma, hypoxia

SPECIAL INVESTIGATIONS

To exclude ... I would do ...

FBC, UE's in delirium, CXR if sepsis, LFT's, gamma GT for monitoring, CT, EEG if seizures, MRI, urine drug screen (other substances).

Other tests if justification:

B_{12}, folate, glucose, ESR, Ca, Po_4, thyroid function tests, albumin, prothrombin time, VDRL, HIV, hepatitis B, C, stool culture for occult blood, neuropsychological assessment if deficits on testing.

- CT – cortical shrinkage, sulcal widening and increased ventricle/brain ratio
- Collateral history and additional information from sources to find out ...
- Role of other professionals – to do what?

Establish a therapeutic alliance

Decrease symptoms using a biopsychosocial model

SHORT-TERM MANAGEMENT OF DETOXIFICATION

Safety

Decrease symptoms using a biopsychosocial approach

- Detox
- Abstinence
- Sobriety

Biological

- Sequelae – monitoring and symptoms
- Advise abstinence and suggest goal may be time limited or indefinite
- Negotiate goals
- Advise safe drinking levels
- Elective withdrawal is usually as an outpatient unless history of:
  Major withdrawal
  Seizure
  Recent head trauma
  Poor social support
  Failed outpatient detox
  Intercurrent illness

Hallucinosis

Treat with benzodiazepines and haloperidol.

Psychological

Discussion, vicarious learning, supportive, self esteem, cognitive behavioural therapy, decrease blame.

Social

Information family, other agencies. AA

LONG-TERM MANAGEMENT

Assessment of motivation to change

Advise period of abstinence and set goals:

- Precontemplation – brief, quick education
- Contemplation – explain, motivation, risk/benefit, loss
- Action – detox, group programme
- Maintenance
- Relapse

Biological

- Monitoring and follow up in outpatients
- Repeat LFTs
- Disulfiram
- Naltrexone

Psychological

Prevent relapse, assertive training.

Marlatt

(1) Identify high risk relapse
(2) understand relapse as event/process factors
(3) Real w/ cues + craving
*   " " social pressure use*
(4) Develop supportive network
(6) Cope w/ -ve emotional states
(7) Plans to interrupt a lapse
*   or relapse*

Family therapy

Part of treatment and in understanding illness and how alcohol is an integral part of their lives and relationships.

Psychotherapy

After abstinence psychotherapy useful, both cognitive behavioural therapy and supportive.

Social

- Family, cohesiveness, increase recovery and decrease blame
- Lack of self care
- Group work, residence

Alcoholics Anonymous 12-step programme

Alcoholics are powerless to overcome the addiction on their own and need the group to help them abstain from alcohol

Group setting is a powerful method to confront denial of illness

Disease model relieves guilt

Abstinent social system and role models

High risk groups

- Armed forces, doctors, journalists
- Alcohol is involved in 25–35% of all suicides and 50–70% of all homicides
- Morbidity – alcohol abuse is associated with many psychiatric and medical disorders

- Care with the elderly who may have alcohol problem – masquerade as organic
- Adolescents abuse alcohol frequently

SEQUELAE OF CHRONIC ALCOHOL ABUSE

Neuropsychiatric disorders

- Intoxication
- Idiosyncratic
- Alcohol withdrawal
- Withdrawal delirium – DT's
- Chronic neuropsychiatric disorders – arise from nutritional deficiencies, gastric malabsorption, hepatic dysfunction associated with chronic alcohol consumption

- Wernicke–Korsakoff
- Cerebral cortical atrophy – diffuse atrophy of frontal cortex
- Cerebellar degeneration – due to Purkinje cells leading to truncal ataxia
- Polyneuropathy – progressive sensory weakness and muscle wasting
- Alcohol myopathy – necrosis of muscle fibres
- Pellagra
- Alcoholic amblyopia – optic nerves blurred – rare
- Marchiafava–Bignami – demyelination of corpus callosum leading to impaired memory and judgement – rare

Alcohol-related brain damage

Wernicke–Korsakoff

- Acute state – carbohydrates worsen the state unless give thiamine with it
- Wernicke's – ataxia, ophthamoplegia, nystagmus, confusion, altered mental state, cerebellar signs, dysarthria
- Korsakoffs – anterograde and retrograde amnesia – decreased insight, apathy and inability to learn, clear consciousness, confabulation
- 20% will recover – treat with thiamine 100 mg orally bd or tds for 3–12 months

Causes of amnestic syndrome

- Thiamine deficiency – alcoholism, malnutrition, carcinoma of stomach, pregnancy, persistent vomiting
- Tumours in the region of the hypothalamus
- Post traumatic
- Subarachnoid haemorrhage
- Infective – syphilis, tuberculosis
- Carbon monoxide poisoning

Frontal lobe dysfunction

- Encountered in alcoholics – circumstantiality, plausibility and weakness of volition – can predispose to relapse
- Ability to diagnose – reason for starting, personality, frontal lobe damage, comorbid depression, social handicap

General treatment – explain goals, include family, comorbidity, alcoholics anonymous, follow-up, self esteem, hope, honesty, open mindedness, willingness.

Alcohol-related dementia

- Impaired problem solving, abstraction, perceptual spatial abilities and new skills and verbal skills
- Large quantities of alcohol more correlation with defects
- Some recovery over 4 months to 5 years but some residual deficit
- Get with continuous drinking, improves with abstinence
- CT shows cortical atrophy and ventricular enlargement

Physical disorders

Systemic disorders:

- Gastrointestinal – oesophagitis, gastritis, hepatitis, pancratitis, Mallory Weiss syndrome, cirrhosis (10–20% develop damage) and sequelae, e.g. varices, jaundice, hepatic encephalopathy, gastrointestinal cancers
- Ascites – salt restriction and bed rest, request medical consult
- Haematological – anaemia, leucopenia, thrombocytopenia
- Cardiovascular – hypertension, cardiomyopathy
- Chronic obstructive airways disease, right heart failure, infection

- Benzodiazepines are metabolized by liver, if oral drugs cannot be used use lorazepam 1–4 mg intramuscularly daily

Management of alcohol related neurological disorder

- Advise abstinence
- Regular thiamine, B vitamins
- Adequate diet
- Physical therapy
- Treatment of alcoholic sequelae, e.g. gastritis, pancreatitis
- Disulfiram – patient must desire it, find it useful and be compliant. No cardiovascular problems, dose of 250–500 mg for 3–5 days. If a patient drinks when taking it they experience flushing, headaches, nausea, vomit, pain, dyspnoea, weakness, dizziness, blurred vision, confusion. Written informed consent
- Experimental agents: naltrexone, acamprosate

Alcohol-induced psychotic disorder

- Auditory hallucinations, voices critical or threatening in clear consciousness
- Treat with benzodiazepines and also nutrition, fluids and antipsychotics if needed

Foetal alcohol syndrome

Mental retardation and microcephaly, craniofacial malformations, limb and heart defects are common, facial abnormalities, irritability in infants, poor coordination, growth deficiencies, hyperactivity in childhood.

Course and prognosis

- Costello found best results if careful patient selection, active therapy, follow up and full use made of supports, e.g. AA
- Relapse is common and needs to be incorporated into the treatment plan

Good prognosis

- Older
- Social support available
- First detox
- Motivated
- Absence of personality disorder in particular antisocial personality traits

AT-RISK SITUATIONS

Alcohol increases the risk to:

- Children
- Partner/spouse
- Self

Increase in domestic violence and accidents. Cycles of violence occur and increased friction in relationships. Cognitive and behavioural strategies are needed to address these issues.

All the above are at increased risk of violence or trauma.

Road traffic accidents/trauma

Increased with alcohol abuse.

Frontal lobe tests

- Generativity – test with verbal fluency, (<13 "c" words in 90 seconds abnormal), write a sentence
- Abstract, proverbs
- Shift sets – pattern reproduction, alternating sequences e.g. fist/palm/side
- Judgement – social setting
- Wisconsin card sort test, trail making tests, frontal release signs, primitive reflexes
- Planning, draw a house, clock
- Primitive reflexes

5.2 ALCOHOL CASE

IDENTIFICATION

30-year-old male who is a labourer, single, currently living with parents.

ISSUES

Management of alcohol dependence and drug dependence.

REFERRAL

via General Practitioner and parents.

PRESENTING COMPLAINT

'Alcohol problem' and methadone.

HISTORY OF PRESENTING COMPLAINT

- Has been drinking alcohol since the age of 15 years when started drinking beer. This was initially at weekends and then progressed to during the week. Last year he started drinking at midday and then earlier in the morning. Has had two fits in the past week. Prior to admission was drinking a bottle-and-a-half of vodka a day. He had time off work due to drinking and would spend days sleeping and drinking
- Had admission last year for detox - 1 week - had a fit. Was treated with diazepam
- Drinking has damaged his social life and also caused him problems at work in that he has been suspended due to drinking
- He has been charged with assault and had several car accidents
- Has attended Alcoholics Anonymous in the past
- He started using drugs at the age of 19 with cannabis, and then progressed onto injecting amphetamines. He started using heroin after a serious road traffic accident when he was awarded $30,000 compensation and bought heroin with it. He could not afford to continue to obtain heroin and so switched to a methadone programme and was using 75 mg prior to admission

PAST PSYCHIATRIC HISTORY

Cut wrists and throat superficially in 1985 as a result of a relationship break up.

RELEVANT NEGATIVES

- No suicidal ideation or intent and not psychotic
- No depressive symptoms

CONSEQUENCES

Biopsychosocial - effect on job, life, parents, health.

CURRENT TREATMENT

Is on diazepam in view of past history of possible fits. Has felt shaky and sweaty.

FAMILY HISTORY

Grandfather was alcoholic and father depressed and used to drink heavily. Youngest of five children.

PERSONAL HISTORY

- Normal development, started to truant from school in his last year. Did not steal as a child. Left school at 16 years of age and did odd jobs. Started smoking cannabis
- Worked as a labourer and was often suspended due to drinking
- Has had several relationships, no one currently. Not experiencing any sex drive over the past 7 months. Living with his parents; on sickness benefit. Outstanding fines owed to court as a result of illegal gun ownership

PAST MEDICAL HISTORY

Nil of note.

CIGARETTES

Smokes one packet a day.

PREMORBID PERSONALITY

Hobbies, interests revolve around drinking, when angry will become physically violent.

MENTAL STATE EXAMINATION

- Appearance and behaviour - dressed casually, good eye contact, no obvious tremor, slightly sweaty
- Speech was coherent and spontaneous
- Mood - anxious
- Affect - euthymic, reactive, full range and mobile
- No suicidal ideation or intent
- Thought content was mainly preoccupied with staying off alcohol and how to get back to work and pay his debts
- No disorder of thought possession
- No abnormal perceptions elicited, not objectively hallucinating
- Cognition - 28/30 on mini-Mental State Examination with abnormalities on short-term memory testing. Digit span was five forwards and four backwards, no frontal lobe abnormalities, no parietal lobe abnormalities, no primitive reflexes
- Insight - recognizes he is an alcoholic and craves alcohol. Has been to Alcoholics Anonymous before and will restart. He wishes to remain on methadone

ON EXAMINATION

- Tattoos, sweaty, no tremor, scars and intravenous injection sites, no enlargement of liver, spider naevi
- Central nervous system - nil abnormal detected, reflexes intact, coordination normal

SUMMARY

In summary he is a 30-year-old man with a 15-year history of increasing use of alcohol. Admitted due to concern from parents and General Practitioner. Has physical complications in the past in that he had fits following an earlier detox. Has an increased compulsion to drink and has had social and legal problems as a result of this. He used to use heroin intravenously but switched to methadone following financial difficulties. He had increased use of alcohol and drugs following a court case. There is some genetic predisposition as his father used to drink heavily. He did have some antisocial traits as a child in that he played truant and had no plans for the future. He has had one episode of deliberate self harm following the break up of the relationship. He has had difficulty in maintaining his job and feels compelled to drink and use drugs. His Mental State Examination shows short-term memory deficit. He appears well motivated to change in that he cannot afford his current habit. He realises it is affecting his life adversely.

ISSUES

- Selective detoxification
- Methadone reduction programme and maintenance
- Short-term memory tests
- Use of disulfiram

DEMENTIA

6.1 DEMENTIA

IDENTIFICATION

Epidemiology: >65 years 5%, >80 years 20%.

REFERRED

Carer, liaison, forensic, General Practitioner, community health centre, self.

ISSUES

Diagnosis, management, carers supports, insight, difficulty, history of behaviour and memory loss, issues pertinent to stage in life cycle, issues pertinent to stage of dementia.

PRESENTING COMPLAINT

Memory loss, behaviour problems, personality, decrease in functioning

Use mnemonic *MAJOR PD*

*M*emory loss – decreased short term and long term memory
*A*bstract thought decreased, Aphasia, Apraxia, Agnosia – four As
*J*udgement decreased
*O*rganicity presumed
*R*ule out depression and
*P*ersonality disorder
*D*ecline in functioning at work and relationships

No neurological signs – degenerative disorder, e.g. Alzheimer's disease

Neurological signs – vascular dementia?

RELEVANT NEGATIVES

Exclude cerebrovascular accident, transient ischaemic attacks, increased blood pressure, alcohol, psychosis, depression, delirium, drug effects (3Ds – Depression, Delirium, Drugs)

ASSESSMENT

- Onset – sudden or gradual?
- NB sudden may be unmasked by death of partner
- Progression – stepwise, abrupt or progressive – depending on cause
- Current difficulties

CONSEQUENCES

- Affect – depressed symptoms, labile, angry, irritable
- Behaviour – disinhibited, aggressive, at risk of abuse
- Problems – relationships at work, social, forensic, navigational
- Severity – current level of functioning – enquire in detail, self care activities, continence
- Find appropriate level of impairment
- Abstract, complex tasks
- Activities of daily living: basic, instrumental, complex

FAMILY HISTORY

Dementia, senility, CVA, multiple sclerosis, psychiatric disorder, depression, drug and alcohol, deliberate self-harm, movement disorders, Huntington's disease, Downs, apolipoprotein E

PERSONAL HISTORY

Usually brief. Ask about exposure to heavy metals, occupation, head injuries, boxing, sexually transmitted diseases.

PAST PSYCHIATRIC HISTORY

Previous admissions, depressive episodes, deliberate self harm.

PAST MEDICAL HISTORY

- Vascular risk – smoke, increased blood pressure, myocardial infarction, atrial fibrillation
- Parkinson's disease, head injury, Downs, iatrogenic, thyroid, gastrectomy (low B_{12}), hypoglycaemia

DRUG AND ALCOHOL HISTORY

Alcohol and possible use of benzodiazepines and anticonvulsants.

PREMORBID PERSONALITY

Coarsening, exaggeration or flattening of traits.

MENTAL STATE EXAMINATION

- Appearance and behaviour – attitude
- Level of activity, apathy, agitation
- Posturing, stereotypies, mannerisms
- Talk, poverty of content, perseveration
- Affect, mood, denial, neglect, psychotic, cognitions consistent with depression, delirium
- Catastrophic reaction
- Failure of new learning

Use mnemonic *CALM FACE*

Consciousness – alert, lethargic, stupor, coma, drowsy

Attention – digits, serial 7s, WORLD

Language – speech naming, repetition, comprehension, reading and writing

Memory – short-term memory, orientation, remote, personal

Frontal lobe tests – alternate hand movements, frontal release signs (palmomental, grasp, snout)

Apraxia, agnosia, astereognosis, aphasia

Construction – figures

Executive functions – general knowledge, abstract, proverbs

ON EXAMINATION

- Cardiovascular system, retina, carotid bruit, blood pressure
- Movement – Huntington's, Pick's (primitive reflexes), Parkinson's (tremor, rigidity, akinesia)
- Thyroid – myxoedema
- Central nervous system – frontal lobe release signs, parietal, upper motor neurone, extrapyramidal side effects
- Primitive reflexes – snout, pout, grasp, glabella, palmomental
- Liver/alcohol stigmata
- Calcium ring
- B_{12} – SACD
- Steele–Richardson syndrome – impaired upward gaze

DIFFERENTIAL DIAGNOSIS

- Psuedodementia (depression, dementia + depression, schizophrenia, anxiety, mania)
- Benign senescent forgetfulness, AAMI age-associated memory impairment
- Delirium – can be demented and delirious
- Amnestic disorder, frontal lobe syndrome, parietal lobe syndrome (Gerstmann)
- Dementia due to general medical condition
- Substance intoxication, withdrawal – causing multiple cognitive deficits
- Mental retardation
- Malingering, factitious

ISSUES

Safety

- Admit only for complications and occasionally for diagnostic clarification.
- Consider deliberate self harm, comorbid depression.

Clarify diagnosis

- Observations and disability
  Inpatient observation – look for depression, diurnal mood variation (typically, am: worse depression, pm: worse dementia), interaction with other patients, activities of daily living
  Look at patients behavioural ability to perform tasks to look after self and person
- Exclude differential diagnosis
- Exclude reversible causes

ASSESSMENT OF MEMORY LOSS IN THE ELDERLY

Memory loss

Benign age-associated.

Pathological memory loss

Functional, depression, mania, anxiety, schizophrenia, hysteria, malingering.

Organic

Acute ?cause delirium, dementia.

Chronic

- Focal
- Dysmnestic syndrome
- Frontal lobe syndrome
- Parietal lobe syndrome
- Dysphasia

Cause of dementia

Potentially reversible

- Thyroid ↓ (or ↑)
- Calcium ↓ (or ↑)
- Folate ↓
- B_{12} ↓
- Tumour – intracranial
- Space-occupying lesion
- Normal pressure hydrocephalus
- Syphilis, AIDS

Irreversible

Cortical

- Degenerative
- Alzheimer's
- Frontotemporal including Picks
- Diffuse Lewy Body disease

Subcortical

- Degenerative
- Vascular dementia
- Parkinson's disease
- Steele–Richardson syndrome

Other

- Alcohol
- Head injury

Nature of deficits

- Language
- Praxis
- Personality

Other pathology

- Sensory
- Physical
- Psychiatric

Patient's assets

Effects on family

CT

- May show cerebral atrophy, focal brain lesions, hydrocephalus
- Help in aetiology of movement disorders, frontal lobe atrophy in Pick's
- Does not give Alzheimer's diagnosis but excludes other causes

EEG

- Slow frontal wave pattern and cortical atrophy on CT in Alzheimer's
- Lesions in the white matter on CT and periventricular white matter hyperintensities with MRI in vascular dementias
- Enlarged ventricles but normal sulci with normal pressure hydrocephalus
- Subcortical degeneration in Parkinson's disease, Huntington's disease

- Collateral history from other sources to verify and provide additional information, e.g. family, other notes, doctors
- Role of other professionals – to do what?
  Domicillary assessment, occupational therapist, physiotherapist, activities of daily living, social work, family therapy, speech therapy

  Care giver support – respite, home helps

Establish therapeutic alliance (if possible)

Decrease symptoms using a biopsychosocial model

SHORT-TERM MANAGEMENT

Aim to keep at home:

Biological

Treat reversible causes, e.g. comorbid depression with:

- SSRI's, SNRI, MAOIs/RIMA, TCA with least anticholinergic side effects, e.g. nortriptiline/desipramine
- Low dose of medication in elderly
- Treat psychiatric symptoms of dementia – antipsychotics

- Consider side effects – use new antipsychotics, e.g. risperidone
- High potency antipsychotics, e.g. haloperidol 0.5–5 mg daily, side effects akathisia and psuedoparkinsonism
- Low potency antipsychotics, e.g. thioridazine 25 mg nocte, side effects: postural hypotension and sedation
- Treatment of dementia with tacrine (TCA) – side effects: nausea, vomiting, diarrhoea, blood dyscrasias. Monitor LFTs and FBC
- Acetylcholinesterase inhibitors – donepezil, rivastigmine, metrifonate

Psychological

Break news, counselling, offer hope, memory aids, support carer, psychoeducation, behavioural strategies.

Social

Occupational therapy, meals on wheels, domiciliary, day centre, mobilise support, carers, financial counselling, enduring power of attorney, wills, general practitioner, social services, work, driving.

MEDIUM-TERM TREATMENT

Biological

Review comorbidity, treatment of behavioural symptoms, psychosis/depression.

Psychological

Ongoing support, carer, remotivation, reminiscence, reality orientation, reinforcement, validation.

Social

Respite day care, behavioural modification.

LATE MANAGEMENT

- Nursing home placement, grief issues, memory loss, cognitive techniques
- Self help Alzheimer's Association

DIAGNOSTIC CRITERIA FOR DEMENTIA OF THE ALZHEIMER'S TYPE Modified with permission from the Diagnostic and Statistical Manual of Mental Disorders, Fourth Edition. Copyright 1994 American Psychiatric Association.

A. The development of multiple cognitive deficits manifested by both

1. Memory impairment (impaired ability to learn new information or to recall previously learned information).
2. One (or more) of the following cognitive disturbances:

- Aphasia (language disturbance)
- Apraxia (impaired ability to carry out motor activities despite intact motor function)
- Agnosia (failure to recognise or identify objects despite intact sensory function)
- Disturbance in executive functioning (i.e. planning, organizing, sequencing, abstracting)

B. The cognitive deficits in (A1) and (A2) cause significant impairment in social or occupational functioning and represent a significant decline from a previous level of functioning.

C. The course is characterized by gradual onset and continuing cognitive decline.

D. The cognitive deficits in (A1) and (A2) are not due to any of the following:

1. Other central nervous conditions that cause progressive deficits in memory and cognition (e.g. cardiovascular disease, Parkinson's disease, Huntington's disease, subdural haematoma, normal pressure hydrocephalus, brain tumour).
2. Systemic conditions that are known to cause dementia (e.g. hypothyroidism, vitamin B_{12} or folic acid deficiency, niacin deficiency, hypercalcaemia, neurosyphilis, HIV infection).
3. Substance-induced conditions.

E. The deficits do not occur exclusively during the course of a delirium.

F. The disturbance is not better accounted for by another axis 1 disorder, e.g. major depressive disorder, schizophrenia.

Early onset <65years

Late onset >65 years

Specify if:

With Delirium
With Delusions
With Depressed Mood
Uncomplicated
With Behavioural Disturbance

AETIOLOGY OF DEMENTIA

DEGENERATIVE

Alzheimer's, Pick's, Huntington's, Creutzfeldt–Jakob, Parkinson's, multiple sclerosis, Wilson's, progressive supranuclear palsy, progressive multifocal leucoencephalopathy.

VASCULAR

Multi-infarct dementia, subarachnoid haemorrhage, ischaemic encephalopathy (Binswanger's disease).

TOXIC

Alcoholic dementia, dialysis, metal toxicity, aluminium, poisons, drugs, e.g. psychotropic drugs and anticholinergic, methyldopa, clonidine, propanolol, anticonvulsants, cimetidine and amantidine.

ANOXIC

Cardiac, respiratory, anaemia, post anaesthesia, carbon monoxide poisoning, post-cardiac arrest.

INFLAMMATORY

Encephalopathies, cranial arteritis, SLE, neurosyphilis, encephalitis.

SPACE-OCCUPYING LESION

Tumour, abscess, haematoma.

METABOLIC

Hepatic, renal.

ENDOCRINE

Myxoedema, hypopituitarism, Addison's, hypo- and hyperparathyroid.

VITAMIN

$B_{1,6,12}$ folate.

NORMAL PRESSURE HYDROCEPHALUS

Ataxia, incontinence, dementia.

TRAUMA

Head injury, punch drunk, child abuse.

EPILEPSY

DISTANT NEOPLASIA

HIV

PREVENTION

No drug has been proven to prevent Alzheimer's disease. However, long-term use of anti-inflammatory drugs and oestrogen replacement therapy in post-menopausal women may have a protective effect. Those at risk of developing Alzheimer's disease (strong family history) should weigh up the risks and benefits of drug treatment.

PROGNOSIS

- Alzheimer's – gradual decline over 8–10 years, progressive disease
- Vascular dementia – onset is sudden, greater preservation of personality, course is stepwise and patchy although some patients have clinical course similar to Alzheimer's
- 90% of Alzheimer's will have psychiatric or behavioural complications during the course of the dementia
- 30% delusions, paranoid ideation, 16% hallucinations, 30% misidentifications syndromes, 5–20% major depressive episode, 20% physical aggression, 20% wandering
- **NB** when diagnose dementia there is a second patient, the family carer. The burden of caring for the patient with dementia is immense. This can be manifest physically, financially, social isolation or psychological distress eg depression, somatic or anxiety symptoms

DISTINGUISH BETWEEN DEMENTIA AND PSUEDODEMENTIA

PSUEDODEMENTIA

- Family aware of history, dysfunction, severity
- Aware of onset of severity
- Date onset with relative precision
- Rapid progression of symptoms and then plateau
- Previous psychiatric dysfunction common
- Cognitive loss complained of
- Detailed complaints of cognitive dysfunction
- Disability emphasised
- Highlight failures
- Communicate sense of distress
- Affective change pervasive
- Loss of social skills
- Behaviour incongruent with severity of cognitive dysfunction
- Answer 'don't know'
- Memory loss, gaps
- Variable performance on tasks

DEMENTIA

- Family often unaware of dysfunction and severity
- Onset known only in broad limits
- Symptoms of long duration
- Symptoms of long course
- Cognitive loss rarely complained of
- Conceal disability
- Delight in accomplishments
- Struggle to perform tasks
- Rely on notes and calendars
- Unconcerned, labile, shallow affect
- Social skills retained
- Attention and concentration faulty, near miss answers frequent
- Memory loss for recent events more severe than remote
- Consistent poor performance on tasks

SIGNS OF CORTICAL DEMENTIA

- Aphasia
- Apraxia
- Agnosia
- Amnesia
- Acalculia

SIGNS OF SUBCORTICAL DEMENTIA

- Slow thinking
- Attention decreased
- Arousal decreased
- Concentration decreased, forgetful, decreased ability to manipulate knowledge
- Motor signs, gait, weakness, incoordination, tremor, reflexes increase, primitive reflexes, posture bowed and extended, gait, tremor, weakness
- Personality change
- Language and parietal lobe function spared

EXTENDED COGNITIVE EXAMINATION

- Attention, concentration (digit span, serial sevens, world backwards), orientation (name day of week, month, year, location)
- Cognitive skills
- Memory
- Reasoning and problem solving

FRONTAL LOBE SIGNS

- Apathy
- Euphoria

- Irritability
- Social inappropriateness
- Lack spontaneity
- Decrease mental and physical activity
- Intellectual impairment
- Poor concentration
- Inability to carry out plans
- Attention deficit
- Sequencing – decreased, slow mental processing
- Executive role, personality, planning, abstraction
- Behavioural control, appropriate
- Disinhibited and euphoric – basal orbital lesion
- Apathy, decreased drive, improved planning – dorsal lateral convexities

FRONTAL LOBE TESTS

- Generativity – test with verbal fluency (<13 'c' words in 90 seconds abnormal), write a sentence
- Abstract, proverbs
- Shift sets – pattern reproduction, alternating sequences e.g. fist/palm/side
- Judgement – social setting
- Wisconsin card sort test, trail making tests, frontal release signs, primitive reflexes
- Planning, draw a house, clock
- Primitive reflexes

TEMPORAL LOBE

- Naming objects, e.g. key, – dominant temporal lobe
- Word finding, reading
- Conversation during interview – receptive language – dominant temporal lobe
- Repetition of words, apple, table, penny – immediate recall – temporal lobes and frontal lobes
- Recall of words – recent memory, name and address, Babcock sentence – hippocampus, thalamus, fornix, mamillothalamic tract
- Long term memory – history, four presidents, last war

DOMINANT PARIETAL LOBE

Gerstmann's syndrome:

- Finger agnosia
- Dyscalculia – simple sums
- Dysgraphia – dictate a sentence and ask patient to write it down
- Right/left disorientation
- Ideomotor apraxia – blow out match, comb hair, simple tasks
- Ideational apraxia – mime putting stamps on letters etc

NON DOMINANT PARIETAL LOBE

Construction apraxia – copy outline of objects.

Dressing apraxia

OCCIPITAL LOBES

- Visual perception defect – cannot name object when camouflaged
- Useful tests – Luria Nebraska, Halstead Reitan, Trail Making test, Bender Gestalt, WAIS R, Wisconsin Card Sorting Test, Ravens Matrices

PERSEVERATION

Occurs in:

- Prefrontal cortex
- Head injury
- Cerebrovascular accident
- Tumours
- Dementias
- Schizophrenia – catatonic

ACTIVITIES OF DAILY LIVING

Basic:
- Bath
- Dress
- Toilet, continence
- Transfer

Instrumental:
- Telephone
- Finances
- Medication management
- Shopping
- Laundry
- Cooking
- Housework

Complex:
- Self direction
- Interpersonal relationships
- Social transactions
- Learning
- Recreation

6.2 DEMENTIA CASE

IDENTIFICATION

75-year-old divorced woman on a pension.

ISSUES

Difficulty in gaining a reliable history due to memory difficulties.

REFERRAL

Admitted 1 week ago via ambulance.

PRESENTING COMPLAINT

'Think hallucinating'.

HISTORY OF PRESENTING COMPLAINT

- Does not remember what was wrong prior to admission to hospital. She thinks she has suffered from bad nerves in the past. She is forgetful and says she does not remember to pay bills
- Has been living on her own

PAST PSYCHIATRIC HISTORY

No admissions - says she has suffered from bad nerves in the past and had some medication. What?

RELEVANT NEGATIVES

Exclude depressive disorder, schizophrenia, drugs and alcohol.

CONSEQUENCES OF SYMPTOMS

Causing disruption to the neighbours and behavioural disturbance.

MANAGEMENT SO FAR

- Admitted and on medication. What?
- On phenytoin - unable to describe type of fits, aura, loss of consciousness, incontinence or when had last fit. Has been on antiepileptic medication since young

FAMILY HISTORY

Parents are both deceased, father was abusive and 'a drunk', mother was a housewife. Four siblings. No family history of any psychiatric disorder apart from alcohol dependence in the father.

PERSONAL HISTORY

Initially lived with her grandparents due to difficulties with her father. Did not enjoy school and left at the age of 14 years to work in a factory. Married and divorced. Two children; one daughter was killed in a road traffic accident over 20 years ago and she is close to the other daughter, although she lives some distance away. They are good friends. Lives in a Housing Commission bedsit and financially is on a pension. Spends her time walking the dog and gardening.

PAST MEDICAL HISTORY

Carcinoma of the bowel - operation in last few months. When?

DRUG /ALCOHOL HISTORY

Nil.

FORENSIC

Nil.

PREMORBID PERSONALITY

Used to enjoy gardening, walks, does get easily hurt on occasion, bottles up stress.

MENTAL STATE EXAMINATION

- Appearance and behaviour - grey haired, elderly woman, glasses, polite, cooperative, tidy, good hygiene, good eye contact
- Speech - little spontaneous
- Mood 'OK', Affect euthymic
- Thought content sparse, no formal thought disorder. No delusions, no disorder of thought possession, not objectively hallucinating and no abnormal perceptions detected
- No obsessive compulsive phenomenon
- Cognition - Mini Mental State Examination testing scored 24/30 with the main abnormalities being disorientation, forgetting the date, unable to recall three items after 3 minutes, difficulties with arithmetic (mental, but written OK)
- There was difficulty in performing frontal lobe testing in that she found fist/palm/side and alternate movements difficult to perform. Alternate sequencing was normal. No primitive reflexes elicited
- No nominal dysphasia. Drawing a clock was normal except for poor spacing. Little general knowledge. Unable to interpret proverbs other than in a concrete way, no apraxia, agnosia or dyscalculia
- Insight - does not understand why she is in hospital

ON EXAMINATION

Examine all systems and exclude relevant negatives, e.g. central nervous system, cardiovascular system.

SUMMARY

A 75-year-old woman probably admitted following a behavioural disturbance. Additionally she suffers memory problems. There is no past psychiatric history of note. She has recently had an operation for cancer and is epileptic. The Mental State Examination reveals paucity of amount and content of speech and difficulty in short term memory, arithmetic, remembering the date and frontal lobe testing, e.g. planning. Possible precipitants to admission may be the operation, medication or behavioural disturbance.

DISCUSSION POINTS

- Delusions and hallucinations are common in people with dementia. 30% of people with Alzheimer's disease will experience delusions, one in six will experience hallucinations
- Management of symptoms and appropriate investigations

SOMATOFORM DISORDERS

7.1 CHRONIC PAIN

IDENTIFICATION

Married with children, employees off sick, life cycle.

REFERRAL

Liaison issues, litigation issues.

HISTORY OF PRESENTING COMPLAINT

Site

- Character
- Onset
- Radiation
- Exacerbation
- Duration

For chronic pain

- Pattern
- Anatomical congruity
- Course over time
- Operant behaviour
- Evidence of gain, symbolism

Behavioural analysis

- Antecedents
- Behaviour
- Consequences

Present level of functioning

- Activities of daily living
- Impairment, disability, handicap
- Sick role

Treatment

- Drug
- Non-drug
- Advantages
- Disadvantages

PAST MEDICAL HISTORY

Somatoform, malingering.

PAST PSYCHIATRIC HISTORY

Any psychiatric disorder, substance abuse.

FAMILY HISTORY

Depression, chronic pain, substance abuse, seen a psychiatrist?

PERSONAL HISTORY

Overachiever, ambitious, workaholic, change with pain symptoms, parental role.

PREMORBID PERSONALITY

Alexithymia.

DRUGS AND ALCOHOL

Used to self medicate.

FORENSIC

Secondary gain, antisocial acts.

SOCIAL

- Operant behaviour, secondary and marital issues
- Litigation common

MENTAL STATE EXAMINATION

Congruity of affect, sick role, secondary depression, suicidal, psychosis.

PHYSICAL

Part of medical assessment.

SOMATIZATION

Use mnemonic *PONSE*

Physical complaints, no panic
Onset <30 years
No organicity
Symptoms – many
Effects, take medications

DIAGNOSTIC CRITERIA FOR SOMATISATION CRITERIA   Modified with permission from the
Diagnostic and Statistical Manual of Mental Disorders, Fourth Edition. Copyright 1994 American Psychiatric Association.

A history of many physical complaints beginning before age 30 years that occur over a period of several years and result in treatment being sought or significant impairment in social, occupational or other important areas of functioning

B. Each of the following criteria must have been met with individual symptoms occurring at any time during the course of the disturbance:

- Pain symptoms – a history of pain related to at least four different sites or functions (e.g. head, abdomen, back, joints, rectum, chest, menstruation, sexual intercourse or during urination)
- Gastrointestinal symptoms – a history of at least two gastrointestinal symptoms other than pain (e.g. nausea, bloating, vomiting other than pregnancy, diarrhoea, intolerance of several different foods)
- Sexual symptom – a history of at least one sexual or reproductive symptom other than pain (e.g. sexual indifference, erectile or ejaculatory dysfunction, irregular menses, excessive menstrual bleeding , vomiting throughout pregnancy)
- Psuedoneurological symptom – a history of at least one symptom or deficit suggesting a neurological condition not limited to pain (conversion symptoms such as impaired coordination or balance, paralysis or localized weakness, difficulty swallowing, lump in throat, aphonia, urinary retention, hallucinations, loss of touch or pain sensation, double vision, blindness, deafness, seizures, dissociative symptoms such as amnesia or loss of consciousness other than fainting)

C. Either (1) or (2):

(1) After appropriate investigation, each of the symptoms in criterion B cannot be fully explained by a known general medical condition or the direct effects of a substance (e.g. drug of abuse, a medication).

(2) When there is a general medical condition the physical complaints or resulting social or occupational impairment are in excess of what would be expected from the history, physical examination or laboratory findings.

D. The symptoms are not intentionally produced or feigned (as in factitious, or malingering).

DIAGNOSTIC CRITERIA FOR UNDIFFERENTIATED SOMATOFORM DISORDER

Modified with permission from the Diagnostic and Statistical Manual of Mental Disorders, Fourth Edition. Copyright 1994 American Psychiatric Association.

A. One or more physical complaints (e.g. fatigue, loss of appetite, gastrointestinal, or urinary complaints).

B. Either (1) or (2):

(1) After appropriate investigation, the symptoms cannot be fully explained by a known general medical condition or the direct effects of a substance (e.g. a drug of abuse, a medication).

(2) When there is a related general medical condition, the physical complaints or resulting social or occupational impairment is in excess of what would be expected from the history, physical examination or laboratory findings.

C. The symptoms cause clinically significant distress or impairment in social, occupational, or other important areas of functioning.

D. The duration of disturbance is at least 6 months.

E. The disturbance is not better accounted for by another mental disorder (e.g. somatoform disorder, sexual dysfunction, mood disorder, anxiety disorder, sleep disorder or psychotic disorder).

F. The symptom is not intentionally produced or feigned (as in Factitious Disorder or malingering).

DIFFERENTIAL DIAGNOSIS

General medical conditions.

Suggestive of somatization disorder:

- Involvement of multiple organ systems
- Early onset and chronic course without the development of physical signs, structural abnormalities
- Absence of laboratory abnormalities characteristic of a general medical condition

Exclude: SLE, hyperparathyroidism, acute intermittent porphyria, Multiple sclerosis. Schizophrenia – multiple somatic delusions need to be differentiated from the non-delusional somatic complaints of individuals with somatization disorders. Hallucinations can occur as psuedoneurological symptoms and must be distinguished from typical hallucinations seen in schizophrenia

- Schizophrenia
- Anxiety disorder
- Panic disorder
- Generalized anxiety disorder
- Mood disorder
- Depressive disorders
- Pain disorder associated with psychological factors, sexual dysfunction, conversion disorder, dissociative disorder
- Hypochondriasis
- Briquets syndrome
- Undifferentiated somatoform disorder
- Factitious disorder with predominantly physical signs and symptoms
- Malingering

HYPOCHONDRIASIS

Use mnemonic *FINDRS*

*F*ear and preoccupation with disease
*I*nterpret physical symptoms as evidence of illness
*N*ormal on examination
*D*espite examination not reassured
*R*ule out panic disorder and psychosis
*S*ix months

DIAGNOSTIC CRITERIA FOR HYPOCHONDRIASIS Modified with permission from the Diagnostic and Statistical Manual of Mental Disorders, Fourth Edition. Copyright 1994 American Psychiatric Association.

A. Preoccupation with fears of having or the idea that one has a serious disease based on the persons misinterpretation of bodily symptoms.
B. The preoccupation persists despite appropriate medical evaluation and reassurance.
C. The belief in criterion A is not of delusional intensity (as in delusional disorder, somatic type) and is not restricted to a circumscribed concern about appearance (as in body dysmorphic disorder).
D. The preoccupation causes clinically significant distress or impairment in social, occupational, or other important areas of functioning.
E. The duration of the disturbance is at least 6 months.
F. The preoccupation is not better accounted for by GAD, OCD, Panic disorder, major depressive episode, separation anxiety or another somatoform disorder.
   - Specify if with poor insight : if for most of the time during the current episode the person does not recognize that the concern about having a serious illness is excessive or unreasonable

DIFFERENTIAL DIAGNOSIS

- General medical condition – early stages e.g. multiple sclerosis, myasthenia gravis, endocrine conditions, e.g. thyroid or parathyroid, systemic lupus erythematosis, occult malignancies
- Somatic symptoms in children
- Health concerns in old age
- Generalized anxiety disorder
- Obsessive compulsive disorder
- Panic disorder
- Major depressive episode
- Separation anxiety
- Somatoform disorder
- Body dysmorphic disorder
- Specific phobia
- Psychotic disorders, e.g. schizophrenia, delusional disorder, major depressive disorder with psychotic features

DIAGNOSTIC CRITERIA FOR PAIN DISORDER Modified with permission from the Diagnostic and Statistical Manual of Mental Disorders, Fourth Edition. Copyright 1994 American Psychiatric Association.

- Pain in one or more anatomical sites is the predominant focus of the clinical presentation and is of sufficient severity to warrant clinical attention
- The pain causes clinically significant distress or impairment in social, occupational or other important areas of functioning
- Psychological factors are judged to have an important role in the onset, severity, exacerbation, or maintenance of pain
- The symptom or deficit is not intentionally produced or feigned (as in factitious disorder or malingering)
- The pain is not better accounted for by mood, anxiety, or psychotic disorder and does not meet criteria for dyspareunia

Pain disorder associated with psychological factors

Psychological factors are judged to have the major role in the onset, severity, exacerbation or maintainance of the pain. (If a general medical condition is present it does not have a major role in the onset, severity, exacerbation or maintainance of the pain.) This type of pain disorder is not diagnosed if criteria are also met for somatization disorder:

- Acute – duration of <6 months
- Chronic – duration of 6 months or longer

Pain disorder associated with both psychological factors and a general medical condition

Both psychological factors and a general medical condition are judged to have important roles in the onset, severity, exacerbation or maintainance of the pain. The associated general medical condition or anatomical site of the pain is coded on Axis III:

- Acute – duration of <6 months
- Chronic – duration of 6 months or longer

Pain disorder associated with a general medical condition

A general medical condition has a major role in the onset, severity, exacerbation or main-tainance of the pain.(If psychological factors are present, they are not judged to have a major role in the onset, severity, exacerbation or maintainance of the pain.) The diagnos-tic code for the pain is based on the associated general medical condition if one has been established or on the anatomical location of the pain if the underlying general medical condition is not yet clearly established, e.g. low back pain, sciatic, pelvic, headache, facial, chest, joint, bone, abdominal, breast, renal, ear, eye, throat, tooth, urinary

MANAGEMENT

Safety

- Suicidality, dangerous drug use, iatrogenic, depression, detox or withdrawal
- Setting – inpatient – severe pain, failed outpatient, large amount of drugs, deliberate self harm

Clarify primary diagnosis

- Observations – a behavioural analysis. Use of pain scales, etc. to provide an assessment of analgesic requirements
- Exclude differential diagnosis
- Collateral history for additional information and verification
- Role of professionals – to do what?
- Often multidisciplinary assessment, e.g. physiotherapist, psychiatry, psychology, rehabil-itation, occupational therapist, anaesthetist

Establish therapeutic alliance

Decrease symptoms using a biopsychosocial model

Use multidisciplinary multimodal rehabilitation approach

Biological

- Low dose tricyclic antidepressants (increase sleep and decrease pain), TENS physio-therapy, hydrotherapy, exercise
- Treat comorbid depression which is common with appropriate antidepressant

Psychological

- Support
- Education

- Cognitive behavioural therapy
- Relaxation skills
- Instill hope, empathy, catharsis, recognition, avoiding triggers, encourage present and future activities

Social

Family support and carer stress, family psychiatry, Any compensation, litigation issues

LONG-TERM MANAGEMENT

- Rehabilitation, occupation and leisure activities, biopsychosocial approach
- Aim to restore to optimum level of functioning
- Use pain scales to show progress

Rehabilitation

- Impairment as a result of illness, secondary impairment and stigma, disabilities and handicaps
- Individual programme – in steps
- Continuity of commitment
- Assessment of individuals – strengths and disabilities

24 hour assessment of all activities

- Self care
- Social relationships
- Work history
- Symptoms and medication
- Individuals own motivations and goals and talents
- Realistic long term goals considering age and disability

Comprehensive approach – multidisciplinary team

- Long term living and work environment
- Functions in environment
- Current skills assessed
- Missing skills
- Resources mobilized
- Survival needs
- Activities for daily living
- Retraining
- Seek job
- Personal fulfilment
- Vocational services

7.2 LIAISON CASE

IDENTIFICATION

Usually on ward or outpatient.

ISSUES

- Detection of depression in the medically ill
- Detection of psychological disorders presenting with somatic symptoms
- Assessment of illness behaviour

DIFFICULTIES

Possible communication with referrer, and others involved with care.

REFERRAL

Via General Practitioner, hospital doctors, nurses.

PRESENTING COMPLAINT

- 'moody, sad'
- 'pain'
- 'aggression'

HISTORY OF PRESENTING COMPLAINT

- Establish any features of depression, establish course and nature of physical illness
- Any comorbid substance abuse
- Effect of illness on family, friends, social and occupational functioning

PAST PSYCHIATRIC HISTORY

Depression, anxiety disorder, substance abuse.

RELEVANT NEGATIVES

Exclude other axis I and II disorders.

CONSEQUENCES

Biopsychosocial - effect on job, life, parents, family, health.

CURRENT TREATMENT

Medical and psychiatric.

FAMILY HISTORY

Depression, pain, patterns of illness behaviour and sick role.

PERSONAL HISTORY

Patterns of illness behaviour and adoption of sick role, role of illness in family, effect of symptoms on relationships.

PAST MEDICAL HISTORY

Often extensive.

CIGARETTES

Smokes one packet a day.

DRUG/ALCOHOL HISTORY

Often comorbid substance abuse.

MENTAL STATE EXAMINATION

- Appearance and behaviour - state of physical health, difficulties with mobility, respiration, gait, hearing, vision, interaction with other staff
- Level of arousal - alert, fearful, hostile, withdrawn, psychomotor retardation, restless, noisy behaviour, responding to hallucinations
- Wandering?
- Confusion - when did it start, in response to what?

- Fluctuating levels of discomfort suggestive of abnormal illness behaviour, i.e. uncomfortable but comfortable when distracted
- Speech - rambling, preoccupation with symptom, physical illness
- Mood/affect - level of mood, anxiety, depression
- Reactivity, range and depth of affect and emotional responses - may be blunted in organic states, detached, bland in somatization, or show inappropriate concern or disability
- Suicidal ideation or intent
- Thought content is usually preoccupied with patients belief about physical symptoms, overvalued ideas or persecutory delusions
- Perceptions - commonly auditory, visual hallucinations when delirious
- Cognitive testing - may have impairment of consciousness, disorientated in time and/or place
- Attention and concentration may be poor, concentration lapses, test with serial 7's and days of week or months of the year backwards
- Short- and long-term memory tests and mini-mental state examination
- Insight - way in which patient explains illness

ON EXAMINATION

Look at medical notes and investigations to date.

ISSUES

Assessment of depressive disorder in the medically ill

- Common reason for referral
- Distinguish depressive disorder from adjustment reactions and define the relationship between depression and medical illness when both are present
- Diagnose depression according to DSM IV criteria, the severity and duration of symptoms are important
- Establish the onset and development of these symptoms
- Presence of somatic symptoms are often indistinguishable from those of the physical disorder

SYMPTOMS OF DEPRESSION IN THE MEDICALLY ILL

*Endicott's criteria (1984), which should be present for at least 2 weeks for a diagnosis of depressive illness.

- Fearful or depressed appearance*
- Social withdrawal or decreased talkativeness*
- Psychomotor retardation or agitation*
- Depressed mood*
- Mood that is non-reactive to environmental events*
- Morning depression
- Marked diminished interest or pleasure in most activities*

- Brooding, self pity, or pessimism*
- Feelings of worthlessness or excessive or inappropriate guilt*
- Feelings of helplessness
- Feeling a burden
- Recurrent thoughts of death or suicide*
- Thoughts that the illness is a punishment
- Frequent crying

Moffic and Paykel describe three patterns of relationship between depression and medical illness:

- Depression as a reaction to the medical disorder and treatment, occurs after illness - two-thirds of depression on medical wards
- Depression that precedes medical illness. Both the depression and illness may start soon after a severe life event e.g. bereavement
- Depressive disorder precedes medical symptoms and may be directly or indirectly responsible for them. Presentation of depression as somatic symptoms is common

DETECTION OF PSYCHOLOGICAL DISORDERS PRESENTING WITH SOMATIC SYMPTOMS

- Is the presenting bodily symptom accompanied by psychological symptoms or other somatic symptoms of anxiety or depression?
- Is the somatic symptom typical of organic disease?
- Previous episode of medically unexplained symptoms
- Precipitation by stress and alleviation by the relief of stress
- Family or past personal history of psychiatric disorder
- Symptoms may respond to psychological treatment when they have failed to respond to medical treatment

DIMENSIONS OF ABNORMAL ILLNESS BEHAVIOUR

- An uncomfortable awareness of bodily events much of the time together with excessive fears and concerns about health and disease
- Relentless search for causes and cures coupled with an inability to accept reassurance from doctors, even when this has been given clearly and on the basis of appropriate investigations
- Adoption of life style around the sick role with repertoire of behaviours to sustain sick role
- Inability to accept the suggestion that non-physical (i.e. psychosocial) factors may be relevant to one's condition
- Disability out of proportion to detectable organic disease
- Reinforcement of illness behaviours by the family, disability payments and healthcare providers

- Inappropriate response to physical disorder - either excessive disability or denial of need for treatment/limitation of activities

MANAGEMENT

Safety and dangerousness

- Be aware of the risk of person to others or themselves
- Nursing special or schedule if necessary
- Move to area where can observe closely

Clarify primary diagnosis

- Observations and disability - ask for reactions of staff
- Exclude differential diagnosis
- Collateral history for additional information and verification. Collect old notes, corroborative history. Discuss with doctors, family, relatives, school, family assessment, ?dysfunction, attitude, conflicts
- Role of professionals – to do what?

SPECIAL INVESTIGATIONS

To exclude ... I would do ...

- Check medical notes for investigations - note if there are any absences or possible causes one would need to exclude
- May make diagnoses of somatoform disorder, pain disorder, hypochondriasis, affective disorders, adjustment disorders, i.e. consider all axis I pathology and axis II for contributing factors

---

Establish a therapeutic alliance

Treatment

- Consider needs of patient using biopsychosocial model and the needs of the staff who may be requesting the consult. Does there need to be intervention with the staff to facilitate management of the patient? Is education of the staff and patient about the illness necessary?
- Remember to give adequate feedback to the referrer as this will also enable clear lines of communication for other referrals and also will be an opportunity to educate about psychiatric diagnoses and management

Patient

- Biological - treat appropriately, e.g. depression with antidepressants - be aware of drug interactions
- Psychological - supportive, educative, may teach specific relaxation techniques, cognitive behavioural strategies

- Social - involvement of family, partner, support mechanisms

LONG-TERM MANAGEMENT

- Ensure follow up with appropriate agency - may be appointments with medical specialist, General Practitioner or liaison follow up
- Biological - monitor drugs and side effects
- Psychological - support, may need more in-depth psychotherapy depending on problem
- Social - maximize supports
- Be available for crises or ensure that numbers and means of contact for a relevant professional are given

SUICIDE AND DELIBERATE SELF HARM

8.1 SUICIDE

IDENTIFICATION

- Older, male, social class I, II, V, bereavement, unemployed, physical illness
- 15% of people with depression and alcohol dependence
- 10% of people with schizophrenia commit suicide

RISK FACTORS – Tuckman and Young

- Age
- Male
- Unemployed
- Separated
- Widowed
- Live alone
- Poor physical health
- Past medical history
- Psychiatric disorder
- Violent attempt
- Suicide note
- Past history of deliberate self harm
- Immigrant, life stresses

Identify risk factors, diminish risk and treat cause.

ASSESS

Social, demographic, clinical factors, suicidal intent, medical seriousness, future plans, after care and support within family situation.

PIERCE SUICIDE INTENT SCORE SCALE

- Assessment of intent
- Circumstances of attempt
- Isolation
- Timing
- Precautions re discovery
- Seek help

- Anticipate death
- Suicide note

SELF REPORT

From patient about lethality, stated intent, premeditated actions and reaction to survival.

RISK

- Likelihood of survival, principles of intervention, diminish cause
- Increased risk in psychiatric patients in acute units is 50 times that of normal population

HIGH-RISK GROUP

- Young, middle aged with affective disorder, schizophrenia
- Women with affective disorders and personality disorders
- Early stages of recovery increase risk as decrease staff vigilance
- Increased risk after discharge – outside factors remain unchanged

Majority of those who suicide talk to someone, e.g. General Practitioner in the previous 3 weeks.

PIERCE SUICIDE INTENT SCORE SCALE

Circumstances related to suicidal attempt

- **Isolation**
  o Somebody present.
  1 Somebody nearby or in contact (as by phone).
  2 No one nearby or in contact.
- **Timing**
  o Timed so that intervention is probable.
  1 Timed so that intervention is not likely.
  2 Timed so that intervention is highly unlikely.
- **Precautions against discovery and/or intervention**
  o No precautions.
  1 Passive precautions, e.g. avoiding others but doing nothing to prevent their intervention (alone in room, doors unlocked).
  2 Active precautions such as locking doors.
- **Acting to gain help during or after attempt**
  o Notified potential helper regarding attempt.
  1 Contacted but did not specifically notify potential helper regarding the attempt.
  2 Did not contact or notify potential helper;
- **Final acts in anticipation of death**
  o None.
  1 Partial preparation or ideation.
  2 Definite plans made (e.g. changes in a will, taking out insurance).
- **Suicide note**
  o None.
  1 Note written but torn up.
  2 Presence of note.

PIERCE SUICIDE INTENT SCORE SCALE

Self report

- **Patients statement of lethality**
  0 Thought what he had done would not kill him.
  1 Unsure if what he had done would kill him.
  2 Believe that what he had done would kill him.
- **Stated intent**
  0 Did not want to die
  1 Uncertain or did not care if he lived or died.
  2 Did want to die.
- **Premeditation**
  0 Impulsive, no premeditation.
  1 Considered act for <1 hour
  2 Considered act for <1 day.
  3 Considered act for >1 day.
- **Reaction to act**
  0 Patient glad that he has recovered.
  1 Patient uncertain whether he is glad or sorry.
  2 Patient sorry he has recovered.

Risk

- Predicatable outcome in terms of lethality of patients act and circumstances known to him
  0 Survival certain
  1 Death unlikely
  2 Death likely or certain
- Would death have occurred without medical treatment?
  0 No
  1 Uncertain
  2 Yes

Suicide intent score

- Low 0–3
- Moderate 4–10
- High 11+

8.2 DELIBERATE SELF HARM

IDENTIFICATION

- Age, sex, marital status, occupation, culture, involuntary or voluntary patient
- Increased in men aged 20–24 years and women aged 15–19 years. Females > males

ISSUES

Safety, therapeutic alliance, prevention of future harm, difficulties and veracity.

REFERRAL

- Accident and Emergency, self, police, other family members
- Overdose is main method combined with alcohol intake

HISTORY OF PRESENTING COMPLAINT

Review suicidal risk, recent context, i.e. loss, life events, insult to self esteem, planning, means, lethality, note, relief at anger, response, relatives, mood sequelae.

Motivation - majority are impulsive acts precipitated by situational crisis.

DIFFERENTIAL DIAGNOSIS

Exclude on axis I depression, psychosis, organic, attention deficit disorder, delirium, dementia. Axis II pathology. Look for secondary gain, malingering.

Use mnemonic *BIAS IRA*

*B*oredom
*I*dentity
*A*nger
*S*uicide threats
*I*mpulsive
*R*elationships
*A*bandonment and affective instability

DIAGNOSTIC CRITERIA FOR BORDERLINE PERSONALITY DISORDER Modified with permission from the Diagnostic and Statistical Manual of Mental Disorders, Fourth Edition. Copyright 1994 American Psychiatric Association.

A pervasive pattern of instability of interpersonal relationships, self image and affects and marked impulsivity beginning by early adulthood and present in a variety of different contexts, as indicated by five (or more) of the following:

1. Frantic efforts to avoid real or imagined abandonment. Note: do not include suicidal or self mutilating behaviour covered in criterion 5.
2. A pattern of unstable and intense interpersonal relationships characterized by alternating between extremes of idealization and devaluation.
3. Identity disturbance – markedly persistent unstable self image or sense of self.
4. Impulsivity in at least two areas that are potentially self damaging (e.g. spend, sex, substance abuse, reckless driving, binge eating) Note: do not include suicidal or self mutilating behaviour covered in criterion 5.
5. Recurrent suicidal behaviour, gestures, or threats or self mutilating behaviour.
6. Affective instability due to a marked reactivity of mood (e.g. intense episodic dysphoria, irritability or anxiety usually lasting a few hours and only rarely more than a few days.
7. Chronic feelings of emptiness.
8. Inappropriate intense anger or difficulty controlling anger (e.g. frequent displays of temper, constant anger, recurrent physical fights).
9. Transient, stress-related paranoid ideation or severe dissociative symptoms.

Use mnemonic *CAR FIRM WAGER*

Conduct disorder
Age 18
Rule out drugs, alcohol, mania and schizophrenia
Fails financial obligations
Impulsive
Risks safety
Monogamous for less 1 year
Work obligations poor
Aggressive
Grounds for repeated arrest
Empathy nil
Repeated lying

DIAGNOSTIC CRITERIA FOR ANTISOCIAL PERSONALITY DISORDER Modified with permission from the Diagnostic and Statistical Manual of Mental Disorders, Fourth Edition. Copyright 1994 American Psychiatric Association.

A. There is a pervasive pattern of disregard for and violation of the rights of others occurring since age 15 years, as indicated by three (or more) of the following:

- Failure to conform to social norms with respect to lawful behaviours as indicated by repeatedly performing acts that are grounds for arrest
- Deceitfulness as indicated by repeated lying, use of aliases, or conning others for personal profit or pleasure
- Impulsivity or failure to plan ahead
- Irritability and aggressiveness as indicated by repeated physical fights or assaults
- Reckless disregard for safety of self or others
- Consistent irresponsibility as indicated by repeated failure to sustain consistent work behaviour or honour financial obligations
- Lack of remorse as indicated by being indifferent to or rationalising having hurt mistreated or stolen from another

Also:

B. The individual is at least 18 years old
C. There is evidence of a conduct disorder with onset before age 15 years
D. The occurrence of antisocial behaviour is not exclusively during the course of schizophrenia or a manic episode

FAMILY HISTORY

Depression, psychosis, drugs and alcohol, deliberate self harm, suicide, antisocial or borderline personality disorder.

PERSONAL HISTORY

Development, early environment – parental separation is common, parental and family relationships, abuse, rejection, school, achievement, peers, occupation, relative duration, quality.

PAST PSYCHIATRIC HISTORY

Personality disorder, depression, psychosis, deliberate self harm, drugs and alcohol.

PAST MEDICAL HISTORY

Renal, diabetes, epilepsy, drugs and alcohol, overdose, head injury, Central nervous system and HIV.

SUBSTANCE ABUSE

Amount, duration and consequences.

SOCIAL

Life events, high number, lonely isolated, inner city unemployed, finances, no close friends.

FORENSIC

Criminal record.

PREMORBID PERSONALITY

Personality disorder, decline in functioning, ego strength

MENTAL STATE EXAMINATION

- Affect, anxious, depressed, inappropriate behaviour, psychosis
- Cognitive – hopelessness, demoralised, anger
- Insight
- Reasons given for act:
    Cry for help, escape from an intolerable situation
    Relief from a state of mind
    To influence others
    Test the benevolence of fate.

ON EXAMINATION

Current overdose and sequelae, evidence of chronic medical illness and drug and alcohol sequelae.

DIFFERENTIAL DIAGNOSIS

Depression, psychosis, panic, personality disorder, substance dependence.

FURTHER ASSESSMENT

Safety

Suicide, inpatient or outpatient monitor and close observations if necessary – if outpatient then relative support and care with drugs, alcohol and signs of substance withdrawal

Clarify diagnosis

- Observations and level of functioning. Regular review of mental state. Be aware of dynamics, e.g. splitting
- Exclude differential diagnosis
  Comorbidity common, e.g. depression. Borderline personality disorder may need containment, boundaries

---

SPECIAL INVESTIGATIONS

As necessary, e.g. drug levels, FBU, UE, LFT, TFT, CA, PO4, glucose

---

- Collateral history for additional information and verification
- Role of other professionals – to do what?

Treat using biopsychological model

Biological

Treat comorbid diagnoses e.g. alcohol dependence or depression.

Psychological

- Crisis counselling and remove stressors
- Empathic listening, support and catharsis, instill hope
- Rally resources and advocacy, practical issues
- Emphasis on problem solving
- Increase psychosocial support and liaise with other agencies

Social

Involvement of other agencies, partners, families.

PROGNOSIS

Depends on age, diagnosis, sex, drugs and alcohol, isolation, life events and hopelessness. Note that each deliberate self harm predicts next deliberate self harm and that 1–2% will suicide.

PREDICTION OF REPETITION

- Previous deliberate self harm
- Previous psychiatric treatment
- Alcohol or drug abuse

- Forensic history
- Personality Disorder especially antisocial
- Social class IV and V
- Unemployment

REPEATED SELF MUTILATION

Types: superficially cut wrists; psychotic patients; seriously suicidal. Many are women and describe increasing tension that is relieved by cutting:

- Young attractive female
- Aged 16–24 years
- Medical/nursing connections in some cases
- Low self esteem
- Comorbid substance dependence (high) and eating disorders
- Poor verbal skills
- Personal history – increased incidence of broken homes and hospitalisation before age 5 years
- Precipitants – recent losses, rejection or relationship difficulties

MANAGEMENT

- Difficulties of team in response to these patients
- Be aware of counter transference issues
- Explore self image and esteem of patient
- Reduce tension by relaxation techniques

PERSONALITY DISORDERS

9.1 BORDERLINE PERSONALITY DISORDER

Use mnemonic *BIAS IRA*

Boredom
Identity
Anger
Suicide threats
Impulsive
Relationships
Abandonment and affective instability

DIAGNOSTIC CRITERIA FOR BORDERLINE PErSONALITY DISORDER Modified with permission from the Diagnostic and Statistical Manual of Mental Disorders, Fourth Edition. Copyright 1994 American Psychiatric Association.

A pervasive pattern of instability of interpersonal relationships, self image and affects and marked impulsivity beginning by early adulthood and present in a variety of different contexts, as indicated by five (or more) of the following:

1 Frantic efforts to avoid real or imagined abandonment. Note: do not include suicidal or self mutilating behaviour covered in criterion 5.
2 A pattern of unstable and intense interpersonal relationships characterized by alternating between extremes of idealization and devaluation.
3 Identity disturbance – markedly persistent unstable self image or sense of self.
4 Impulsivity in at least two areas that are potentially self damaging (e.g. spend, sex, substance abuse, reckless driving, binge eating) Note: do not include suicidal or self mutilating behaviour covered in criterion 5.
5 Recurrent suicidal behaviour, gestures, or threats or self mutilating behaviour.
6 Affective instability due to a marked reactivity of mood (e.g. intense episodic dysphoria, irritability or anxiety usually lasting a few hours and only rarely more than a few days.
7 Chronic feelings of emptiness.
8 Inappropriate intense anger or difficulty controlling anger (e.g. frequent displays of temper, constant anger, recurrent physical fights).
9 Transient, stress-related paranoid ideation or severe dissociative symptoms.

IDENTIFICATION

Female more than male.

ISSUES

Axis II versus axis I depression, comorbidity, spectrum of drug and alcohol abuse, psychotic symptoms.

Management

Therapeutic alliance, transference and counter transference, self destructive behaviour.

DIFFICULTIES

Veracity and rapport.

REFERRAL

Self, Accident and Emergency, deliberate self harm, police.

HISTORY OF PRESENTING COMPLAINT

- Depression, drugs and alcohol, overdose, decrease in ego strength cohesion
- Onset and course, chronic instability
- Severity – decompensation, brief psychotic episode

Consequences

Suicide, deliberate self harm, self mutilation, dysfunctional domains, relationships, parent, work, forensic misconduct.

FAMILY HISTORY

Increased affective disorders, drugs and alcohol and antisocial personality disorder.

PERSONAL HISTORY

- Longitudinal, brain damage in childhood
- Studies show that 60% of men and 30% of women with Borderline personality disorder have impaired rating on the Luria Nebraska Neuropsychological tests
- Sexual and physical abuse as child, many job losses, interrupted education, broken marriages

PAST PSYCHIATRIC HISTORY

Comorbid drugs and alcohol, mood disorders, substance related, eating disorder, bulimia, post traumatic stress disorder, attention deficit hyperactivity disorder, other personality disorder.

PAST MEDICAL HISTORY

Hepatitis, cirrhosis.

PREMORBID PERSONALITY

Use mnemonic *HERMI*. Often comorbid personality disorders

Habitual defences
Egoistic strength
Relationships
Mood stability
Impulsivity/identity

FORENSIC

Driving charges (reckless driving).

SOCIAL

Support, life events, finances, accommodation.

MENTAL STATE EXAMINATION

Unstable affect, mood, lability, suicidal ideation, low self esteem, brief psychotic symptoms, drug intoxication and withdrawal, ideas of reference, hallucinations, hypnogogic hallucinations.

DIFFERENTIAL DIAGNOSIS

- Mood disorder
- Histrionic personality disorder
- Schizotypal personality disorder
- Paranoid personality disorder
- Narcissistic personality disorder
- Antisocial personality disorder
- Dependent personality disorder
- Due to change in general medical condition, e.g. central nervous system
- Chronic substance use, e.g. cocaine
- Identity problem

ON EXAMINATION

Evidence of self harm, lacerations, liver damage, needle tracks.

MANAGEMENT

Safety and dangerousness

- Mental Health Act and setting
- Crisis admission – united team approach, contract, time limited, limit setting
- Medical treatment as required

Clarify diagnosis

- Observations and disability. Regular review of mental state
- Exclude differential diagnosis

SPECIAL INVESTIGATIONS

To exclude ... I would do ...
FBC, UE, LFT, TFT, urine and drug screen

- Collateral history from another source to verify information and to find out what ...
- Role of other professionals – to do what?

Establish a therapeutic alliance

Decrease symptoms using a biopsychosocial model

Biological

- Target, symptom, subject relief, treat underlying depression (SSRIs, SNRI, TCA, MAOI), be aware of potential of overdose, neuroleptics if psychotic symptoms; anxiety and anger, self destructive behaviour; role of benzodiazepines, treat alcohol intoxication or withdrawal
- Lithium is mood stabilizer, clozapine for impulsive rage.

Psychological

- Rapport, alliance, empathy, respect, supportive treatment, self esteem, limit setting, review safety, outpatients, psychotherapy, consult, review, social advocacy, accommodation and welfare
- Staff issues, shared burden of care, supervision, support

LONG-TERM MANAGEMENT

Biological

Assess mood state – and treat appropriately (see above).

Psychological

Supportive.

Social

Case management, multidisciplinary team, advocacy, staff support and shared care.

Prognosis

- Anticipated difficulties, drugs and alcohol, deliberate self harm, suicide, splitting
- Gunderson's model is one of the individuals relationship to the major or primary object – this is the person to which the borderline currently has a significant relationship
- If the person is supportive then the primary symptoms are depression and dysphoria
- If the object is perceived as frustrating then anger, manipulation, and devaluation of the major object occur and suicidal gestures
- If the object is absent then the person may feel abandoned, experience depersonalization, devaluation, ideas of reference or frank brief psychotic episodes occur. Impulsive, acting out behaviour represents an effort to ward off and manage the loneliness and subsequent disintegration and restore self esteem

Individual treatment

Studies show that 50% of borderline personality disorders drop out in 6 months and 75% in the first year. Only 1 in 10 complete a course of psychotherapy. Counter transference is strong – despair, rage, etc. Supervision necessary.

Long-term psychotherapy

The aim is to overcome resistance in establishing a relationship with the primary object (the therapist) and understanding and dealing with the fluctuations once an ongoing therapeutic relationship has been established. Regression occurs easily

Projective identification – may cause counter transference problems if the therapist is unaware that the patient is unconsciously trying to coerce the therapist to a particular type of behaviour.

Splitting is a defence mechanism which causes patient to love or hate environment/person.

Behavioural therapy

Decreases impulsivity

Social skills training

With videotape feedback

Management of psychiatric crises

- Self destructive acts
- Identify the nature and cause of disruption
- Intervene to restore calm and integration
- Hospitalize – acute crises to restore milieu
- Intensive hospitalization – receive intense psychotherapy on individual and group basis – 1 year – then discharge to half way house and support etc.

9.2 ANTISOCIAL PERSONALITY DISORDER

Use mnemonic *CAR FIRM WAGER*

Conduct disorder
Age 18
Rule out drugs, alcohol, mania and schizophrenia
Fails financial obligations
Impulsive
Risks safety
Monogamous for less 1 year
Work obligations poor
Aggressive
Grounds for repeated arrest
Empathy nil
Repeated lying

DIAGNOSTIC CRITERIA FOR ANTISOCIAL PERSONALITY DISORDER   Modified with permission from the Diagnostic and Statistical Manual of Mental Disorders, Fourth Edition. Copyright 1994 American Psychiatric Association.

A. There is a pervasive pattern of disregard for and violation of the rights of others occurring since age 15 years, as indicated by three (or more) of the following:
- Failure to conform to social norms with respect to lawful behaviours as indicated by repeatedly performing acts that are grounds for arrest
- Deceitfulness as indicated by repeated lying, use of aliases, or conning others for personal profit or pleasure
- Impulsivity or failure to plan ahead
- Irritability and aggressiveness as indicated by repeated physical fights or assaults
- Reckless disregard for safety of self or others
- Consistent irresponsibility as indicated by repeated failure to sustain consistent work behaviour or honour financial obligations
- Lack of remorse as indicated by being indifferent to or rationalising having hurt mistreated or stolen from another

Also:

B. The individual is at least 18 years old
C. There is evidence of a conduct disorder with onset before age 15 years
D. The occurrence of antisocial behaviour is not exclusively during the course of schizophrenia or a manic episode

IDENTIFICATION

3% male, 1% female.

ISSUES

Legal, forensic.

FAMILY HISTORY

- Risk that the disorder develops in first-degree relatives is greater than the risk for the general population
- Adoption studies indicate both a genetic and environmental risk, some familial association between antisocial personality disorder, histrionic personality disorder, and somatization

PERSONAL HISTORY

Deprivation as child, harsh upbringing and use of aggression, work record poor, relationships erratic, lack of intimacy, lack of loyalty and promiscuous behaviour.

ALCOHOL AND SUBSTANCE ABUSE/DEPENDENCE

High.

PAST PSYCHIATRIC HISTORY

Conduct disorder as child.

FORENSIC HISTORY

Positive, did what? Consequences?

MENTAL STATE EXAMINATION

Suicide threats.

DIFFERENTIAL DIAGNOSIS

- Substance related disorder
- Other personality disorders, e.g. narcissistic, histrionic, borderline, paranoid
- Schizophrenia
- Mania
- Adult antisocial behaviour

- Diagnosis – can have abnormal EEG, immature pattern

MANAGEMENT

Safety

Clarify diagnosis

- Observations and disability
- Exclude differential diagnosis. To exclude ... I would do
- Collateral history from other source to verify information and find out what ...
- Role of other professionals – to do what?

Establish a therapeutic alliance (often difficult)

Decrease symptoms using a biopsychosocial model

Biological treatments

- Lithium, propanolol, anticonvulsants, e.g. carbamazepine, may help for patients with impulsive and explosive behaviour
- No clear effective treatment
- Comorbidity with schizophrenia, mania, drugs and alcohol

Psychological

- Individual psychotherapy has not been successful in treating antisocial individuals
- Groups – self-help groups can be helpful if person feels among peers and there are firm limits set and the group can look at the patients fear of intimacy
- Family therapy – useful and provides support for the family
- Therapeutic communities – closed highly structured, residential treatment programmes

Social

- Management in the hospital and therapeutic community, drug and alcohol treatment, crisis intervention
- Contract of the management and limit setting, use trained nursing staff
- Identify factors causing aggressive behaviour, e.g. head injury, drugs and alcohol, job loss, and those which prolong and worsen it
- Coping strategies

Discussion Issues

- Problem of therapy – sabotage, premature termination, aggressive stance, counter transference reactions
- Forensic issues, dangerousness and staff issues
- Increased risk of suicide, homicide, accidents
- Course – less evident as get older

FORENSIC

10.1 DANGEROUS PATIENTS

IDENTIFICATION

Young male, marital status, occupation and culture.

ISSUES

Safety, compliance and comorbidity.

DIFFICULTIES

Veracity.

REFERRAL

Police, detention, relatives.

HISTORY OF PRESENTING COMPLAINT

1. Ideational features, e.g. violent thoughts.
2. Affective – anger, destructive rage.
3. Behavioural features – psychotic, agitated, family arguments.
   - Psychotic phenomena, e.g. delusions – persecutory, grandiose, jealous, erotomania
   - Command hallucinations?
   - Details of any violent act
   - Homicidal
   - Non psychotic – increased arousal, impulsive anger, aggressive thoughts, jealousy, panic, fear, recurrent rejection, self righteousness, no evidence of remorse, sense of vengeance, need for suspiciousness
   - Depression – deliberate self harm, homicidal
   - Drugs and alcohol – amphetamines and PCP
   - Victim known, context, provokes, harm, psychotic, premeditated, attention, remorse, isolated act

RELEVANT NEGATIVES

Drug and alcohol, command hallucinations, suicidal ideation, compliance, treat if psychotic.

ASSESSMENT

OFFENDER PLUS VICTIM + CIRCUMSTANCE = OFFENCE

1. Type of violence.
2. Degree – excessive.
3. Quality – bizarre.
4. Disinhibiting factors – drugs.
5. Behaviour after the offence – humane feelings, egocentric actions.

FAMILY HISTORY

Increased family history of psychosis, violence, aggression and antisocial personality disorder.

PERSONAL HISTORY

- Early environment, development and parental care, issues of control and abuse, loss, relationship discord, repeated maladaptive pattern of behaviour, learning attentional problems at school and achievement, peers
- Interpersonal relationships – response to rejection
- Conduct disorder – lying, cheating, stealing, fighting and poor occupation, exploitative, substance abuse
- Previous offences, aggressive behaviour, childhood deprivation, abnormal personality traits, paranoid, impulsive, inability to cope with stress, delay gratification and poor self control

PAST PSYCHIATRIC HISTORY

- Psychosis – type and content of delusions and hallucination
- Morbid jealousy
- Treatment, compliance
- History of violence in past setting
- Drugs and alcohol

PAST MEDICAL HISTORY

Head injury, birth trauma, temporal lobe epilepsy, cerebral insult, hypoxia, secondary to overdose and alcohol, drug sequelae and HIV, hepatitis.

PREMORBID PERSONALITY

- Self assessment, self confidence and esteem, habitual mood, obsessional, perfect, impulsivity, anger, aggression, identity, coping mechanism/strengths
- Antisocial, Borderline, Paranoid, sense of entitlement, urge to redress wrong

SOCIAL HISTORY

Risk taking, violent lifestyle, loss of relatives, employment, financial difficulties.

FORENSIC HISTORY

- Convictions, assault, grievous bodily harm, malicious wounding
- Past record of violence predicts violence

MENTAL STATE EXAMINATION

- Arousal, hypervigilance, suspicious, agitation, voice, tone, eye contact, pacing, paranoid, misinterpretations, fearfulness, irritability, frustration, catatonia, psychotic symptoms, persecutory delusions, drug intoxication, cognitive testing, insight, judgement
- Psychotic? Command hallucinations or instructions
- Does he conform? Emotional rapport, capacity for empathy
- Cognitive – organic brain lesion?

ON EXAMINATION

- Drug intoxication and stigmata, drug withdrawal, recent trauma, head injury, neurological signs (soft), increased arousal, delirium, fever, skull fracture

DIFFERENTIAL DIAGNOSIS

- Psychotic illness – schizophrenia, schizophreniform, delusional, paranoid
- Affective disorder
- Drug-induced
- Organic – delirium, drugs, alcohol, withdrawal states, dementia, epilepsy, brain injured
- Antisocial personality disorder, borderline and paranoid personality disorder
- Impulse control disorder
- Adjustment disorder with a disturbance of conduct
- Obsessive compulsive disorder

MANAGMENT ISSUES

Safety

- Past violence is the best indicator
- Obtain history of violence, e.g. arrest record, prior violence, driving record, victims, means of violence used or planned for future use, planned premeditation of violence, sense of futility, e.g. 'there is no future', precipitants to violence and 'Why now?'

Restraint

Observe and document

- Nursing observations regularly
- May need to use haloperidol, droperidol or diazepam intravenously
- Referral precautions
- Use of Mental Health Act
- Immediate setting, acute, locked, specialist inpatient facility
- Trained staff-to-patient ratio
- Milieu will decrease stimulation and reassurance with clear limits and intervention

Clarify diagnosis

- Collaborative, police, forensic.
- Exclude medical emergencies, differential diagnosis

SPECIAL INVESTIGATIONS

FBC, UE's, glucose, LFT, drug screen, paracetamol levels, stimulants, PCP, CXR, SXR

Progress in custody

- Rebel or conform, self control or manipulate system?
- Ability to participate in psychotherapy and transference issues

PREVENTION

- Risk and precautions
- Clear explanations, firm boundaries, repeated explanations
- Availability of appropriate trained staff
- Rule out triggers and other disturbances
- Decrease stimuli – non confrontational and remove disturbance
- Future support

Biological

- Oral sedation if accepting
- Benzodiazepine sedation for the non delirious patient
- For intramuscular sedation use midazolam and for intravenous, diazepam. Parenteral droperidol is more sedating than haloperidol and associated with fewer dystonic reactions but it may have more effect on blood pressure and pulse rate and has a shorter half life than haloperidol
- Zuclopenthixol acetate is useful for sedation and antipsychotic treatment for up to 3 days in some patients but is associated with extrapyramidal side effects. Avoid if suspect NMS
- Anticholinergic drugs to be available if signs of dystonia ensure prn benztropine 1–2mg prescribed when parenteral drugs are administered
- Flumazenil a benzodiazepine antagonist should be available when giving intravenous benzodiazepines

SHORT-TERM MANAGEMENT

- Depends on diagnosis
- Custodial care if violence not psychotically driven
- Forensic issues – warn potential victim
- Discharge planning – establish treatment and contact relations
- Follow up – community care - community treatment order
- Liaise with family and police, confidentiality
- Monitor compliance – depot and establish means of early intervention crisis service for the family
- Deal with factors around the violence, e.g. poor social skills, impulsivity, drugs and alcohol, family conflict, poor compliance
- Forensic issues and ethical issues, restraining order, write report, confidentiality – duty to protect the public – Tarasoff doctrine

OFFENCE

Bizarre violence, drugs and alcohol, lack remorse, continuing denial, lack of provocation, failure to consider alternative to violence.

PREDICTORS OF HOMICIDE

- High degree of intent to harm
- Victim
- Frequent and open threats
- Concrete plan
- Access to instruments of violence
- History of loss of control
- Chronic anger, hostility, resentment

- Enjoy watching or inflicting harm
- Lack of compassion
- Self view as a victim
- Resentful of authority
- Childhood brutality
- Decreased warmth and affection
- Early loss of parent
- Firesetting and bedwetting as a child
- Prior acts of violence
- Reckless driving

RISK INCREASES OF HOMICIDE

- Disruptive family life
- Poor functioning
- Unsuitable lifestyle
- Lower socio-economic status
- Unemployed
- Illiterate, drop out
- Poor housing, overcrowding
- Isolation, withdrawal, loner
- Chronic alcohol abuse
- Past psychiatric treatment
- Family history of violence
- Anxious, moody
- Poor self image
- Aggression
- Need for violence
- Becomes constrictive under stress, acts out in socially unacceptable ways
- Marked, lose contact with reality
- Unable to use resources available or recognise help is available
- Multiple arrest history
- Thoughts of homicide
- Weapons available and planning on use

SOCIAL

- Frustration, direct provocation, aggressive models, e.g. on the television, disinhibits, desensitisation
- Situational determinants, sexual arousal, pain, hormone, genetic

DIFFERENTIAL DIAGNOSIS FOR HOMICIDE

- Schizophrenia
- Drug and alcohol
- Organic brain syndrome
- Epilepsy
- Intermittent explosive disorder
- Antisocial personality disorder

DISORDERS ASSOCIATED WITH AGGRESSION Modified with permission from the Diagnostic and Statistical Manual of Mental Disorders, Fourth Edition. Copyright 1994 American Psychiatric Association.

- Mental retardation
- Attention deficit and hyperactivity disorder
- Conduct disorder
- Cognitive disorders, e.g. delirium, dementias
- Psychotic disorder, e.g. schizophrenia, psychotic disorder not otherwise specified
- Mood disorders, due to general medical conditions
- Substance induced mood disorder
- Intermittent explosive disorder
- Adjustment disorder with disturbance of conduct
- Personality disorders – paranoid, antisocial, borderline, narcissistic
- Axis V codes – childhood, adolescent or adult antisocial behaviour

Characteristics

- Majority of the adults who commit aggressive acts are likely to do so against persons they know, usually family members. Homicide most common if know each other
- Episodic decompensation may occur in persons who ingest large quantities of alcohol

ASSESSMENT OF DANGEROUSNESS

Offence

- Type
- Frequency
- Attitude to it and victim
- Premeditation
- Victim characteristics and precipitating factors

Social factors

- Relationships, work, family
- Mental status
- Employment
- Finance

Biological

- Alcohol, drugs
- Cerebral dysfunction

Psychological

- Mental illness
- Personality, overcontrol, undercontrol
- Impulsivity, capacity for concern
- Sadism
- Attitude to self, family, minority groups

MOVEMENT DISORDERS

11.1 DRUG-INDUCED MOVEMENT DISORDERS

DEFINITION

Involuntary movements and abnormalities of muscle tone caused by current or previous medication use. Due to blockade (e.g. Parkinsonism) or upregulation (e.g. TD) of dopamine receptors.

IDENTIFICATION

Old age, tardive dyskinesia, known psychiatric illness.

HISTORY OF PRESENTING COMPLAINT

- Symptoms – may have a variety of presentations. Tremor, bradykinesia, rigidity, as manifest by shuffling gait, change in writing, soft speech, difficulty swallowing, involuntary movements, stiffness, odd posture (often noticed more by relatives than the patient). Parkinson's disease may be mistaken for early depression due to reduced facial expression.
- Drug history – duration and type of drug important. Drugs ceased, even years previously, may still be relevant. Neuroleptics, antiemetics, drugs for vertigo, oral contraceptive pill (rarely causes chorea).

PAST PSYCHIATRIC HISTORY

Schizophrenia, mannerisms, stereotypies, neuroleptics, tardive dyskinesia.

PAST MEDICAL HISTORY

Conditions of relevance, e.g. head injury, CVA, Parkinson's disease, MS, CO poisoning, liver problems (?Wilson's disease).

FAMILY HISTORY

Psychiatry, medical. Huntington's disease has variety of presentations

PERSONAL HISTORY

- Effect of movement disorder on functioning
- Psychosocial issues
- Functional assessment, e.g. self care, activities of daily living, mobility

MANAGEMENT

Safety

Consider person is at risk.

Clarify diagnosis

- Observations and disability, inpatient observation
- Exclude differential diagnosis
  Main treatable causes are Wilson's ($\uparrow$Cu) drugs and rarely increased manganese
  Identify main disability:
  ?Parkinsonism, ?chorea, ?tremor, ?combination
  Drug-induced extrapyramidal 'syndromes', e.g. akathasia and Parkinsonism
  Identify suspected drug(s)
  Cease suspected drug(s) and replace with drug(s) least likely to cause problem if clinically necessary
  Consider alternative causes of the above

SPECIAL INVESTIGATIONS

To exclude ... I would do ...

FBC, ESR, LFT, Cu, B$_{12}$, Mn, folate, drug, HIV, VDRL, TFT, CT, MRI, genetic, CT or MRI (if suspect Huntingtons)neurological examination, urine heavy metal screen

---

- Collateral history to provide additional and verify information
- Role of professionals – to do what? Refer to neurologist if diagnostic or therapeutic uncertainty

Establish a therapeutic alliance

Decrease symptoms using a biopsychosocial model

- Treat once diagnosis established
- Try to avoid using a second drug to treat extrapyramidal symptoms

SPECIFIC EXTRAPYRAMIDAL SYNDROMES

DYSTONIA

- An increase in muscle tone (usually focal) often with persistent attitude or posture. May be task specific

- Occurs in 10% of patients initiating therapy with antipsychotics

TORTICOLLIS (type of dystonia)

A contraction of the neck muscles causing the head to be drawn to one side and usually rotated so that the chin points to the other side. Retrocollis, opisthotonus, oculogyric crisis are also dystonias involving neck muscles. Usually develops within 2 days of the treatment with neuroleptics and produces dystonias in the first 12–24 hours. Most common with the high potency neuroleptics, e.g. haloperidol and fluphenazine. Overall incidence of the acute dystonic reactions following the initiation of the neuroleptic medication is about 5%. Male > female by 2:1. Dystonia is more common between 20 and 45 years of age.

Treatment – acute dytonic reactions are responsive to immediate administration of anti-cholinergeric agent. Typical treatment may include an intramuscular or intravenous injection of benzotropine.

PARKINSONISM

See chapter 11.2

AKATHISIA

Subjective desire to be in constant motion with an inner sense of restlessness. Most common manifestation is shuffling the feet while sitting. Wide range of prevalence of akathisia reported in those receiving neuroleptic medication (20–75%). With slow release or depot neuroleptics the onset of akathisia occurs sooner within 1–4 days. Development of akathisia appears to be dose-dependent.

- Akathisia is the most resistant of the extrapyramidal symptoms to effective treatment
- First choices – lower the dose of neuroleptic or switch to one of a lower potency neuroleptics
- Second choice – benztropine 2 mg tds, diphenhydramine 25 mg tds, propranolol 20 mg tds
- Third – amantidine 100 mg tds
- Fourth – benzodiazepines
- Rate using the Barnes or the Prince Henry Akathisia scales

DIFFERENTIAL DIAGNOSIS OF NEUROLEPTIC-INDUCED ACUTE AKATHISIA

- Akathisia of Parkinson's disease and iron-deficiency anaemia
- SSRI medications
- Medication-induced movement disorders not otherwise specified
- Neuroleptic-induced tardive dyskinesia
- Agitation seen in other axis I disorders, e.g. depressive episodes, manic episodes, GAD, schizophrenia, other psychotic disorders, attention-deficit/hyperactivity disorder, delirium, dementia, substance intoxication, substance withdrawal

TARDIVE DYSKINESIA (TD)

Hyperkinetic movement disorder that occurs after prolonged treatment with neuroleptic medication. Characteristically refers to repetitive chewing movements, lip smacking and tongue rolling. This can be transiently suppressed when requested but rapidly returns. There may be associated choreo-athetoid movement of hands or feet. The symptoms are due to up-regulation of dopamine receptors after prolonged blockade. Stress exacerbates movements.

Usually does not develop before 2 years of treatment but can occur sooner (3–6 months). If movements resolve within 3 months the prognosis is usually good.

- Prevalence of TD varies widely with the mean prevalence 24%
- Prevalence affected by populations studied, institutional/non-institutional, medication status, age group, methodological issues

Risk factors for TD include:

- Age
- Sex, females at slightly greater risk (1.7:1)
- Neuroleptic medications – consider duration of use, drug dose and type, high versus low potency, typical versus atypical, age at initiation of dose, drug holidays, history of extrapyramidal side effects or akathisia
- Anticholinergic drugs (worsen the manifestations)
- Lithium (unlikely)
- SSRI/TCA (can produce a TD-like syndrome)
- Diagnosis of schizophrenia (with negative symptoms), affective disorder, mental retardation, organic brain dysfunction
- Concurrent general medical disease

Other risk factors include:

- Smoking
- Diabetes
- Alcohol/drug dependence
- Dental status (ill-fitting dentures, edentulous)
- Ethnicity
- Familial-genetic factors

DIFFERENTIAL DIAGNOSIS OF NEUROLEPTIC-INDUCED TARDIVE DYSKINESIA

- Huntington's disease
- Wilson's disease
- Sydenham's (rheumatic) chorea
- Systemic lupus erythematosus
- Thyrotoxicosis
- Heavy metal poisoning
- Ill-fitting dentures
- Dyskinesia due to other medications, e.g. L-dopa, bromocriptine, amantidine

- Spontaneous dyskinesias
- Neuroleptic-induced Acute Dystonia
- Neuroleptic-induced Acute Akathisia

PREVENTION

- Prevention is the best strategy. Advise patients to report symptoms when commence medication
- Use agents with less risk of developing TD, e.g. chlorpromazine, thioridazine, clozapine
- Avoid drug holidays, anticholinergic drugs
- Use the lowest dose possible to control symptoms and maintain patient
- Use atypical neuroleptics
- Treat risk factors if possible, e.g. smoking, dental problems, alcohol use, diabetes, anticholinergic medication
- Use Abnormal Involuntary Movement Scale AIMS every 3 months to evaluate TD. (see chapter 2.2)
- Could also use videotape ratings and instrumental ratings, e.g. electromechanical instruments, frequency counts, ultrasound, accelerometers, vocal assessments, EMG
- Evaluate patients regularly who are receiving antipsychotic medication
- Attend to dentition and dental hygiene

TREATMENT

- Stop medication if possible
- Reduce the dose of neuroleptic and switch to those less likely to cause movement disorders
- Natural history is a fluctuation course with spontaneous remissions and exacerbations
- 50% show improvement in 5–10 years
- A number of drugs can be tried, e.g. antidopaminergic agents, tetrabenazine, GABAergic, (valproate, baclofen, benzodiazepine), antiadrenergic (propanolol, clonidine)

LITHIUM TOXICITY

- Fine lithium tremor seen at start of lithium treatment
- Benign and does not cause difficulty
- Self limiting usually. If continues treat by eliminating caffeine, relaxation techniques, reduce oral dose of lithium slightly, try propranolol
- Coarse tremor is sign of intoxication and occurs in association with other symptoms of neurotoxicity, e.g. ataxia, dysarthria, visual disturbances, mental confusion
- Discontinue lithium, determine lithium levels and determine what corrective measures are necessary, e.g. stomach emptying, emesis, NaCl administer, correct fluid balance, and dialysis. Note that lithium toxicity can occur with serum lithium levels that are only slightly above the reference range

NEUROLEPTIC MALIGNANT SYNDROME

Definition

Catatonic state associated with fever, obtundation, muscle rigidity and unstable vital signs seen in patients taking neuroleptic agents. Estimated incidence is 1 in 1000, but the phenomena is under-recognised. Mortality used to reach 15–20% but is less now due to greater recognition. It is common in patients taking depot agents.

Aetiology

- Male > female, age <40 years, physical factors are present, triggers for NMS include: dehydration, physical exhaustion, heat stress, nutritional deficiencies, concurrent organic mental disorder
- Fluphenazine is the most commonly implicated along with haloperidol
- Increase risk with dose, and number of injections
- Associated with schizophrenia, affective disorders
- Symptoms – fever, muscle rigidity, altered consciousness, autonomic instability
- Additional symptoms – tremor, dyskinesia, akinesia, oculogyric crisis, opisthotonus, chorea, dysarthria, sialorrhoea, respiratory complications
- Early course – usually in first 2 weeks of treatment or after increase of drug
- It can occur at any time during antipsychotic drug use. Labile vital signs, elevated blood pressure precede symptoms of 3–5 days. Lasts for up to 30 days. Progresses rapidly within 24–72 hours

SPECIAL INVESTIGATIONS

- Creatinine phophokinase increased
- Leucocytosis
- EEG
- Liver function tests (LFT's)
- FBC, CPK, urea, nitrogen, Cr, UE, TFT, Mg, LP, EEG, CT, toxicology, lithium
- Develop rhabdomyolysis therefore urine contains myoglobin/blood

DIFFERENTIAL DIAGNOSIS OF NEUROLEPTIC MALIGNANT SYNDROME

- Malignant hyperthermia – muscle rigidity, fever develop rapidly after exposure to inhalational anaesthetics
- Acute lethal catatonia – sustained agitation that progresses to hyperpyrexia, withdrawal, catatonia, cardiovascular collapse and death
- Heat stroke
- Central nervous system infection, e.g. encephalitis, tetanus
- Other disorders – hyperthermia, central anticholinergic syndrome, akinetic mutism
- Hypertonic states, e.g. hysterical rigidity, decorticate or decerebrate rigidity, tetany, strychnine poisoning, abrupt withdrawal of dopamine depleting agents
- Symptoms due to other neurological or general medical conditions
- Other psychotropic medications

TREATMENT

- Withdraw agent, start or continue anti-Parkinsonian treatment
- Supportive measures – antipyretics, aspirin
- Dantrolene – intravenously 2–3 mg over 10–15 min
- Bromocriptine – 2.5–10 mg tds, increased to 60mg/day
- Alternatives – amantidine 200–400 mg/day, benzodiazepines, L-dopa, carbidopa
- Correct hydration, vitamins, nutritional supplements when possible, monitor renal function
- Treatment of the NMS – adjunctive use of benzodiazepines
- After several weeks of recovery patients may be retreated with antipsychotic medication cautiously usually with a lower potency antipsychotic medication than the precipitating agent or clozapine (although this can also cause NMS)
- Complications – renal (rhabdomyolysis with myoglobinuria), cardiac arrest or MI with pulmonary oedema, pulmonary embolism, hypoxia, anterior tibial syndrome, other complications, e.g. sepsis, hepatic failure, DIC

11.2 PARKINSONISM

Parkinsonism is a cluster of symptoms (Akinesia, Rigidity, Tremor). The commonest cause is idiopathic Parkinson's Disease.

IDENTIFICATION

40–70 years old, more common in men, 1% of population >50 years.

REFERRAL

GP, family, patient.

HISTORY OF PRESENTING COMPLAINT

- Early symptoms may be difficult to perceive
- Usually asymmetric
- Patient often presents as result of "stiffness" due to side effects of medication
- Anticholinergics may cause presentation for confusion or hallucinations
- Use mnemonic *ART*

  *A*kinesia
  *R*igidity
  *T*remor

AKINESIA

- Expressionless face, poverty and slowness of movement, soft monotonous voice
- Handwriting becomes smaller (micrographia)

RIGIDITY

Stiffness, cogwheeling.

TREMOR

- Resting tremor, 'pillrolling' at 3 Hz

Cognitive changes

Secondary depression or dementia.

Expressionless face often mistaken for depression.

MEDICATIONS

Which? How long? On/off phenomenon.

Ldopa and dopamine agonists for rigidity.

Anticholinergics for tremor.

Ask about medication side effects, e.g. postural hypotension, incontinence, confusion.

CONSEQUENCES

- Effect on ability to care for self, effect on carers, family, etc
- Functional assessment of independence
- Incontinence, falls, aspiration

FAMILY HISTORY

Depression, dementia, tremor.

PERSONAL HISTORY

Any psychosocial issues resulting from illness.

PAST MEDICAL HISTORY

- Vascular risk factors – hypertension, obesity, cholesterol, diabetes, family history of ischaemic heart disease, peripheral vascular disease
- Medication – antipsychotic, antiemetic, intravenous drug use

PAST PSYCHIATRIC HISTORY

Depression, dementia, family history of Parkinson's disease.

MENTAL STATE EXAMINATION

Signs of depression, dementia, Mini Mental State examination.

ON EXAMINATION

- Walk the patient. Look for loss of postural control with retropulsion, stooped posture, shuffling gait, tendency to 'rush' forwards. Freezing
- Work from the periphery in towards the centre
- Tremor, frequency, tone, cogwheel/lead pipe, BP – postural drop (exclude autonomic neuropathy – Shy Drager syndrome), downward gaze and convergence (exclude pro-

gressive supranuclear palsy Steele–Richardson syndrome), excess sweating, drooling, seborrhoea, dysarthria, pout, primitive reflexes, grasp, palmomental, glabella tap (sign of frontal lobe involvement)
- Full neurological examination

MANAGEMENT

Safety

Reactive depression.

Clarify diagnosis

- Observations and disability, inpatient observation rarely required unless complications
- Exclude differential diagnosis

DIFFERENTIAL DIAGNOSIS

Idiopathic Parkinson's Disease

Due to other primary CNS diseases

Alzheimer's, CVA, progressive supranuclear palsy, diffuse Lewy body disease

Corticobasal degeneration

Familial tremor (fine quality manifest during volitional movements and disappears at rest), tremor from cerebellar disease

Paucity of movements in patients with retarded depression, normal pressure hydrocephalus, frontal lobe damage (head injury, Pick's)

Drug-induced, e.g. phenothiazine effects, reserpine, haloperidol, pimozide causing a masking of face, stiffening of limbs, lack of arm swing, fine tremor and mumbling speech, antiemetics

Toxins – Mn, Cu, CO

Primary mental disorder, e.g. depression

- Collateral history to provide additional and verify information.
- Role of professionals – to do what?

SPECIAL INVESTIGATIONS – limited value as clinical diagnosis

To exclude ... I would do ...

- FBC to exclude increased white cell count, UE for Cr, LFTs, ESR
- If necessary B_{12}, folate, HIV, VDRL
- Exclude vascular risk factors

- CT or MRI to look for vascular changes in the basal ganglia and atrophy of caudate (Huntington's)
- SPECT – corticobasal degeneration

Establish therapeutic alliance

Decrease symptoms using a biopsychosocial model

Treatment

- Dopaminergic agents, e.g. L-dopa (Sinemet, Madopar) mainly beneficial for rigidity and akinesia
- Used in conjunction with benztropine, procyclidine. L-dopa has side effects, give in divided doses, combine with peripheral dopa-decarboxylase inhibitor to prevent its rapid destruction in the blood and permit the control of symptoms more quickly and with a lower dose. Early side effects include nausea and hypotension
- May get on/off phenomenon over long-term
- Anticholinergic agents mainly beneficial in tremor – in conjunction with L-dopa – side effects: dry mouth, blurred vision, constipation, mental slowing, confusional states, hallucinations, impairment of memory, postural hypotension
- Amantidine – an antiviral agent helps reduce rigidity, hypokinesia and also tremor. Side effects include oedema of legs
- Bromocriptine – use cautiously – longer duration of action than L-dopa and causes nausea and vomiting less often
- Selegeline – mode of action unclear
- Newer dopamine agonists, e.g. pergolide

Treat psychiatric manifestations

- Often comorbid depression in Parkinson's disease which needs treating, e.g. tricyclic antidepressants, SSRIs
- Difficulties in distinguishing PD from depression due to earliest motor manifestations of PD, e.g. loss of agility, loss of facial expression, sense of slowness – look for depressed mood and anhedonia
- Prevalence of depression in PD is 51% in clinic/hospital based studies and 32% in population studies. There is no relationship between the age of onset, duration of illness, and the presence of depression in PD
- Profile of depressive features include elevated levels of dysphoria, pessimism re: the future, irritability, sadness and suicidal ideation, little guilt, self-blame, feelings of failure or punishment. Prominent psychiatric manifestations suggest alternate diagnosis e.g. Alzheimer's, diffuse Lewy Body disease
- Mania is rare and usually associated with excess dopaminergic treatment
- Psychosis can be the result of dopaminergic stimulation – reduce the antiparkinsonian medication if possible.
- Clozapine – less extrapyramidal side effects. May be useful in the clinical treatment of tremor – at low doses (see chapter 2.2)

- Personality changes – nil specific – may get increased irritability as disease progresses with its disability
- Cognitive impairment and dementia
  Restrictive deficits in executive function, visuospatial function and memory. Dementia is more common with late onset PD (see chapter 6.1 for details of cognitive assessment).

DIFFICULTIES

- Management of the on/off phenomenon – attempt to even out dopamine levels throughout the day
- Strategies include decrease dose, increase frequency of medication
- Consider use of ECT for depression
- Tremor may be hard to treat – may need to resort to unilateral thalamotomy
- Rigidity – consider pallidotomy

11.3 GILLES DE LA TOURETTE SYNDROME

IDENTIFICATION

Disruption in family, male>female, onset prior to age 18 years, 0.5/1000 prevalence.

HISTORY OF PRESENTING COMPLAINT

- Are the tics voluntary or involuntary?
- Can the person suppress the movements with concentration and if so for how long?
- Onset of tics – motor and vocal of variable severity, waxing and waning course
- Average age of onset is 7 years
- Initial tics are in the face and neck, e.g. grimacing, puckering of forehead, raise eyebrow, blinking of eyelids, winking, wrinkling of the nose, trembling nostrils, twitching mouth, displaying the teeth, biting of the lips, extrude tongue, licking, protract lower jaw, nod, jerk, shake head, twist neck, look sideways, head roll
- Arms and hands jerk, clench fists, body and lower extremities, shrug shoulders, shake foot, knee, toe, peculiarities of gait, body writing, jumping, squatting, forced touching
- Respiratory and GIT, hiccup, sigh, yawn, sniffing, blow through nostrils, whistling inspiration, exaggerated breathing, belching, sucking or smacking sounds and clearing the throat, smelling, spitting
- Prodromal behavioural symptoms, e.g. irritable, attention difficulties, poor frustration tolerance
- Most common initial symptom is eyeblink tic then head tic or facial tic. More complex motor and vocal symptoms emerge several years after the initial symptoms. Coprolalia starts in early adolescence in about one-third of cases. Mental coprolalia may also occur
- Echolalia (the imitation of sounds or words of others) and echopraxia (the imitation of movements or actions of others) occur in 11–44% of patients
- Palilalia (the repetition of the last word or phrase in a sentence or the last syllable of a word uttered by the patient) occurs in 6–15% of patients

ASSOCIATED SYMPTOMS

- Obsessions and compulsions, hyperactivity, distractibility, impulsivity are also common
- Social discomfort, shame, self consciousness and depressed mood frequently occur
- Attention deficit hyperactivity disorder, learning disorder, obsessive compulsive disorder are all associated

AGGRAVATED BY

Anxiety, stress, boredom, fatigue and excitement.

RELIEVED BY

Sleep, alcohol, orgasm, fever, relaxation or concentrating on an enjoyable task.

CONSEQUENCES

- Social, academic and occupational functioning may be impaired due to rejection by others or having tics in social situations. Severe cases may interfere with daily activities
- Rare complications include physical injury, blindness due to retinal detachment (from head banging or striking oneself), orthopaedic problems (from knee bending, jerking, head turning), and skin problems (from picking)

DIAGNOSTIC CRITERIA FOR TOURETTES DISORDER Modified with permission from the Diagnostic and Statistical Manual of Mental Disorders, Fourth Edition. Copyright 1994 American Psychiatric Association.

- Both multiple motor and one or more vocal tics have been present at some time during the illness, although not necessarily concurrently
  (A tic is a sudden rapid, recurrent, non-rhythmic stereotyped motor movement or vocalization)
- The tics occur many times a day (usually in bouts) nearly every day or intermittently for >1 year, and during this time there was never a tic-free period of >3 consecutive months
- The disturbance causes marked distress or significant impairment in social, occupational or other important areas of functioning
- The onset is before age 18 years
- The disturbance is not due to the direct physiological effects of a substance (e.g. stimulants) or a general medical condition (e.g. Huntington's disease or postviral encephalitis)

MEDICATIONS

What helped? What has been used in the past successfully and unsuccessfully?

FAMILY HISTORY

Genetic basis, often strong family history.

PERSONAL HISTORY

- Effect of disorder on development. Details of developmental milestones, level of attainment
- Psychosocial issues. Difficulties due to behaviours

PAST MEDICAL HISTORY

Seizures, birth, ischaemic risk factors, febrile convulsions, hypoxia, trauma, cerebral insult.

PAST PSYCHIATRIC HISTORY

Obsessive compulsive disorder.

MENTAL STATE EXAMINATION

Depressive symptoms, obsessive compulsive symptoms, tics and mannerisms.

PHYSICAL EXAMINATION

Full neurological examination, e.g. chorea, dystonia, torticollis, dysphonia, dydiadochokinesis, postural abnormalities, reflex asymmetries, motor incoordination, nystagmus, and unilateral Babinski reflexes. Localize signs, e.g. use startle and test with clap, clicking of fingers, etc. Tone, rigidity, spasticity

MANAGEMENT

Safety

Consider if person is depressed and at risk.

Clarify diagnosis

- Observations and disability, inpatient observation
- Exclude differential diagnosis

DIFFERENTIAL DIAGNOSIS

- Abnormal movements that accompany general medical conditions
  For example, Huntington's disease, stroke, Lesch–Nyhan disease, Sydenham's chorea, multiple sclerosis, post viral encephalitis, head injury
- Direct effect of substance, e.g. neuroleptic medication
- Athetosis – slow irregular twisting of muscles in the distal portions of legs and arms
- Chorea – irregular, jerky movement of muscles. Choreic movements are more rapid and involve more muscle groups than do athetotic movements
- Hemiballismus – intermittent, violent, unilateral flinging movements of the extremities
- Dystonia – Task specific – characterized by sustained contraction of both agonist and antagonist muscles, producing abnormal postures of the head, neck, limbs or trunk. Rigidity continued resistance to passive stretching of the muscles
- Myoclonic movements are brief shock-like muscle contractions that may affect parts of muscles or muscle groups but not synergistically
- Hemifacial spasm – irregular repetitive unilateral movements of the limbs
- Medication-induced movement disorder not otherwise specified, e.g. methylphenidate may exacerbate a pre-existing tic disorder
- Stereotypic movement disorder
- Pervasive developmental disorders
- Obsessive compulsive disorder – distinguish tics from compulsions
- Schizophrenia – catatonic behaviour
- Chronic motor or vocal tics

SPECIAL INVESTIGATIONS

To exclude ... I would do ...

FBC, ESR, LFTs, B$_{12}$, folate, drug, HIV, VDRL, TFT, CT, MRI, EEG. Blood and urinary copper levels, serum caeruloplasmin, Kayser Fleisher rings (to exclude Wilson's).

Some MRI scans have found minor abnormalities in the basal ganglia. PET and SPECT have demonstrated metabolic and perfusion abnormalities in the basal ganglia and frontotemporal areas with special reference to the putamen.

- Collateral history to provide additional and verify information
- Role of professionals – to do what? Clarify role

Establish therapeutic alliance

Decrease symptoms using a biopsychosocial model

Biological

- Haloperidol, may need anticholinergic agent
- Pimozide

- Sulpiride
- Clonidine
- SSRIs used to treat obsessive compulsive aspects of GTS

Psychosocial management

- Education re disease
- Supportive psychotherapy
- Counselling
- Advice to patient and family, teacher re disorder
- Individual tuition, extra explanation and time in class and exams

COURSE AND PROGNOSIS

Chronic life long disease with relative remissions and exacerbations.

PSYCHODYNAMIC

12.1 INSIGHT AND DEFENCE MECHANISMS

The assessment of this is often poor. It is an important part of the Mental State Examination.

Questions to ask are:

- Does the patient see themselves as ill?
- Does the patient feel in need of help?
- Is the patient compliant?
- Does the patient deny illness?
- Does the patient see it in terms of physical or mental illness?
- Do they need treatment?

LEVELS OF INSIGHT

- Is there complete denial of the illness?
- Are they aware that they are sick and deny it also?
- Are they aware that they are ill but attribute it to external factors?
- Are they aware that illness is due to something unknown in the patient?
- Do they have intellectual insight, i.e. admit that they are ill but do not apply knowledge to their experience?
- Do they have true insight of their motives and behaviour?
- Do they have psychological insight?

It is comments about insight that often give examiners an idea of a candidate's maturity and sophistication in being able to probe into the meaning of the experiences for the patient.

PSYCHODYNAMIC FORMULATIONS

Consider the following headings:

- Think of the context of the defence style
- Is there a psychological precipitant?
- Is there a symbolic meaning?
- What is the personality style?
- What is the life stage?
- Ego characteristics
- Object relations

- Self structure
- Transference/counter transference issues

CHARACTERISTICS OF THE EGO

- Work and relationship patterns
- Reality testing
- Impulse control
- Judgement
- Psychological mindedness of patient
- Defensive functioning of ego - desires/wants/fears/wishes/fantasy
- Relationship of ego to superego

OBJECT RELATIONS

- Information about the patients interpersonal relationships in childhood, the transference in the interview and relationships outside the doctor/patient relationship
- Try to establish what old object relationship is being repeated and the role of the patient in it. Level of maturity of the object relations is important

THE SELF

- Durability and cohesiveness of self
- Self esteem
- Maturity of patients self objects
- Boundaries of self/object

DIFFERENT CATEGORIES WITH A PARTICULAR FORMULATION STYLE

- Illnesses
- Neurotic disorders, personal style, includes anxiety disorders, OCD/personality, cluster C
- Disorders of self - cluster B's

Illnesses

These include schizophrenia, bipolar affective disorder, depression, eating disorders, other psychoses. Can usually use stress/diathesis or biopsychosocial paradigms. Obviously precipitants, symbolic meaning of symptoms, defensive style has some importance but perhaps more weight should be added to issues such as coping style/Erikson stage (especially with respect to identity/intimacy/generativity issues).

Does the axis I diagnosis account for the severity of the patients functional impairment or do features on axis II contribute to a lower level of functioning?

Use Erikson's life stages to discuss life cycle:

- Trust versus mistrust
- Autonomy versus shame
- Initiative versus guilt
- Industry versus inferiority
- Identity versus role diffusion
- Intimacy versus isolation
- Generativity versus stagnation
- Integrity versus despair

Neurotic disorders Cluster C's

Classical/object relations psychoanalytical model provides an appropriate theoretical under-pinning, i.e. drive/defence. Try to establish characteristic defences, core conflicts, object relations.

OBSESSIVE COMPULSIVE PERSONALITY DISORDER

DIAGNOSTIC CRITERIA FOR OBSESSIVE-COMPULSIVE PERSONALITY DISORDERS Modified with permission from the Diagnostic and Statistical Manual of Mental Disorders, Fourth Edition. Copyright 1994 American Psychiatric Association.

A pervasive pattern of preoccupation with orderliness, perfectionism, and mental and interpersonal control at the expense of flexibility, openness and efficiency, beginning by early adulthood and present in a variety of contexts, as indicated by four (or more) of the following:

- Is preoccupied with details, rules, lists, order, organization or schedules to the extent that the major point of the activity is lost
- Shows perfectionism that interferes with task completion (e.g. is unable to complete a project because his/her overly strict standards are not met)
- Is excessively devoted to work and productivity to the exclusion of leisure activities and friendships (not accounted for by obvious economic necessity)
- Is over conscientious, scrupulous and inflexible about matters of morality, ethics or values (not accounted for by cultural or religious identification)
- Is unable to discard worn out or worthless objects even when they have no sentimental value
- Is reluctant to delegate tasks or to work with others unless they submit exactly to their way of doing things
- Adopts a miserly spending style toward both self and others; money is viewed as something to be hoarded for future catastrophes
- Shows rigidity and stubbornness

Typical obsessional defences used, e.g. intellectualization, rationalization and isolation of affect, reaction formation and undoing.

Within individual therapy modifications include strategies such as seeking impressions and emotive reactions to events rather than just detailed factual accounts and then link the emotional meaning rather than accepting the isolation of ideas from emotions. This requires an active therapeutic stance which activates the dominance/submission core conflicts. The working through via the transference is a key feature of the psychoanalytically oriented approach.

Other Cluster C personality disorders look at the issue of dependency with the vulnerable self which is threatened in various interpersonal situations, particularly close ones.

Avoidant personality disorder have a vulnerable self which desires closeness but avoids it for 'fear of rejection'.

Dependent personality disorder cling to others and fear they will lose them.

Disorders of self Cluster B's

- Self psychological approach
- Defensive style is crucial as is the assessment of sense of self, structure, esteem, boundaries
- Identity disturbance with emptiness and abandonment - lack of integrated sense of self.
- Constant presence of people required to maintain a sense of integration and to ward off emptiness and abandonment. Immature methods of dealing with primitive rage and anxiety
- Need to have some understanding as to how a sense of identity develops in early childhood in the first 6 months. Lack of integration of self. Use of behaviours is to maintain a view of themselves. These patients depend on continuing validation of their subjective state from another person. If this does not occur it is perceived as abandonment. Impulsive behaviours which are potentially self-harming are ways to remedy the emptiness.

DIAGNOSTIC CRITERIA FOR BORDERLINE PERSONALITY DISORDER Modified with permission from the Diagnostic and Statistical Manual of Mental Disorders, Fourth Edition. Copyright 1994 American Psychiatric Association.

A pervasive pattern of instability of interpersonal relationships, self image and affects, and marked impulsivity beginning by early adulthood and present in a variety of different contexts as indicated by five or more of the following:

1. Frantic efforts to avoid abandonment. Note: do not include suicidal or self mutilating behaviour covered in criterion 5.
2. Pattern of unstable and intense interpersonal relationships characterized by alternating between extremes of idealization and devaluation.
3. Identity disturbance - markedly persistent unstable self image or sense of self.
4. Impulsivity in at least two areas that are self damaging (e.g. spending, sex, substance abuse, reckless driving, binge eating). Note: do not include suicidal or self-mutilating behaviour covered in criterion 5.
5. Recurrent suicidal behaviour, gestures, threats or self mutilating behaviour.
6. Affective instability due to a marked reactivity of mood (e.g. intense episodic dysphoria, irritability, or anxiety usually lasting a few hours and only rarely more than a few days).
7. Chronic feelings of emptiness.
8. Inappropriate intense anger or difficulty controlling anger (e.g. frequent displays of temper, constant anger, recurrent physical fights).
9. Transient stress - related paranoid ideation or severe dissociative symptoms.

DEFENCES USED IN DISORDERS

- Affective disorder uses repression, denial and internalizes anger
- Mania uses projection
- Schizophrenia uses splitting and autistic fantasy
- Paranoid uses denial, projection, splitting and rationalization
- Paranoid personality disorder uses projection, projective identification
- Schizoid and schizotypal use social inhibition and restrict affect and denial
- Antisocial personality disorder uses impulsivity, aggression, failure of object relations to develop basic trust, poor conscience, displacement
- Borderline personality disorder uses splitting, projective identification, idealization, fear of abandonment, turn of hate into self, ego dysfunction and identity disturbance
- Histrionic personality disorder uses regression, dissociation, identification, conversion, denial, externalization
- Narcissistic personality disorder uses entitlement, grandiosity and empathic failure, separation and individuation phase, passivity, depressive features, self image, ego ideal, omnipotence
- Obsessive compulsive personality disorder uses isolation, undoing, reaction formation, intellectualization, rationalization.
- Avoidant personality disorder uses avoidant and inhibition, condensation, displacement, aggression
- Hysteria uses denial, projection, identification and repression
- Anxiety uses regression, autistic fantasy
- Panic uses regression
- Agoraphobia uses projection/displacement - repressed hostility projected onto the environment as it is seen as dangerous
- Phobias use avoidance and displacement
- Post-traumatic stress disorder uses regression, repression, denial, undoing
- Somatoform disorders uses dissociation
- Substance dependence uses oral, dependent, denial, ambivalent
- Eating disorders uses separation/individuation issues, transient food, ambivalent relationships

DEFINITIONS OF DEFENCES

- Repression is a refusal to recognize internal reality
- Denial is a refusal to recognize external reality
- Projection is an attribution of unacknowledged feelings to others
- Distortion is a grossly reshaping of external reality to suit inner needs
- Reaction formation is a way of feeling and behaving in a way that is opposite of unacceptable instinctual impulses
- Displacement - redirect feelings
- Dissociation - interruption of integrated functions of consciousness, memory, identity or perception of the environment

- Depersonalization - alteration in perception or experience of self so that one feels detached from and as if one is an outside observer of ones mental processes or body (feeling as if you are in a dream)
- Projective identification - unwanted aspects of self deposited on another person, person is aware of feelings and misattributes them as a justifiable reaction to other person
- Acting out - direct expression of unconscious impulse in order to avoid awareness of accompanying affect
- Intellectualization - way of thinking, rather than feeling about desires
- Sublimation - indirect expression of instincts without adverse consequences
- Suppression - intentionally avoid disturbing problems, wishes and feelings
- Splitting - the positive and negative fantasized relationships remain alternatively in consciousness with the alternative dissociated
- Isolation - separation of idea from affect, individual copes by being unable to experience cognitive and affect components of an experience simultaneously as affect is kept from consciousness
- Affiliation - help, from others support, share problems, do not make them responsible
- Transference - repetition of past which is inappropriate to the present, transfer unconscious memories into consciousness
- Counter transference - therapists attitude to patient, therapeutic alliance, adult patient, transference neurosis
- The model of projective identification is helpful in understanding counter transference. Due to the various provocative behaviours in the patient the psychiatrist may start to feel like a projected self or object representation of the patient

Awareness of feelings can help the psychiatrist to understand the nature of the patient's internal object world and problems in the patients interpersonal relationships

DEFENCE MECHANISMS (ACCORDING TO VAILLANT'S CLASSIFICATION)

NARCISSITIC DEFENCES

- Denial
- Distortion
- Primitive idealization
- Projection
- Projective identification
- Splitting

IMMATURE DEFENCES

- Acting out
- Blocking
- Hypochondriasis
- Identification
- Introjection
- Passive aggressive behaviour

- Projection
- Regression
- Schizoid fantasy
- Somatization

NEUROTIC DEFENCES

- Controlling
- Displacement
- Dissociation
- Externalization
- Inhibition
- Intellectualization
- Isolation
- Rationalization
- Reaction formation
- Repression

MATURE DEFENCES

- Altruism
- Anticipation
- Asceticism
- Humour
- Sublimation
- Suppression

13 MANAGEMENT OF ANXIETY IN THE EXAM SITUATION

PREPARATION

It is obvious that it is important to work out what the examiners are expecting of you and what skills one is supposed to convey in the examination. These skills may be maturity, sophistication, leadership and diplomacy, as well as the ability to synthesize and integrate clinical information and provide clinical diagnoses and treatment plans.

Empathy and interaction with the patient will also be assessed either directly or indirectly by the examiners when meeting the patient (usually while the candidate is writing up their formulation or treatment plan).

Practising in a simulated exam situation is useful as well as having mock examiners asking questions of you.

Most of your preparation will be from your working life and the clinical cases encountered every day.

Try to plan a scheme for answering questions in a logical manner and also for assessing patients so that you do not leave out any vital pieces of information.

Aim to see patients you are not currently working with under exam conditions so that you refresh yourself about the particular problems of that group of patients. It is often the practical issues in management that are lacking in the exam, and it is knowledge of these that convinces an examiner that you have managed a patient of this kind before.

PRIOR TO EXAM

- Remain as calm as possible. Remember some anxiety in this situation is normal and will enhance your performance although excessive anxiety can be detrimental
- Prepare adequately
- Keep physically fit as well as mentally agile
- Aim for a healthy lifestyle, reduce alcohol consumption
- Remember that management of stress in the exam situation is also assessed - performance will diminish if you have too much anxiety
- Practise slow breathing techniques or imaginal desensitization
- Practise relaxation techniques
- Visit the exam site prior to the exam

The post graduate clinical examinations is often the first occasion when candidates 'fail to satisfy the examiners'. It is important to keep this in perspective as no examination system is infallible and the nature of a clinical exam means that there is an element of luck involved in terms of examiners and patients, even with the most thorough preparation. Candidates who are in this position should not give up but use the extra time before the next examination to rethink their approach to psychiatric cases and management, and take the time to learn about areas which are less usual but may be of use in clinical practice. Remember you are equipping yourself for a lifetime of psychiatric practice and the best person to prepare you for that is yourself with your own awareness of your limitations.

Good luck!

14 MNEMONICS

AGORAPHOBIA

FEDSA

Fear place or situation
Escape
Difficult
Symptoms develop
Avoidance

ANOREXIA NERVOSA

RABID

Refusal to maintain body weight – 15%
Amenorrhoea
Behaviours – weight losing behaviours
Intense morbid fear of further weight gain
Disturbance in the way weight and size are perceived

ANTISOCIAL PERSONALITY DISORDER

CAR FIRM WAGER

Conduct disorder
Age 18
Rule out drugs/alcohol, mania and schizophrenia
Fails financial obligations
Impulsive
Risks safety
Monogamous for less than 1 year
Work obligations poor
Aggressive
Grounds for repeated arrest
Empathy nil
Repeated lying

BORDERLINE PERSONALITY DISORDER

BIAS IRA

Boredom
Identity
Anger
Suicide threats
Impulsivity
Relationships
Abandonment and affective instablity

BULIMIA

BORCEN

Binge – twice a week for 3 months
Over concern with body shape and image
Restricted eating or no eating between binges
Control of eating diminished
Engages in bulimic behaviour
Normal body weight

COGNITIVE TESTING

CALM FACE

Consciousness – alert, lethergic, stupor, coma, drowsy
Attention – digit span, serial 7's, WORLD
Learning – speech naming, repetition, comprehension, reading and writing
Memory – short term memory, orientation, remote, personal
Frontal lobe tests – alternate hand movements, frontal release signs (palmomental, grasp, snout)
Apraxia, agnosia, astereognosis, aphasia
Construction – figures
Executive function – general knowledge, abstract, proverbs

DELIRIUM

FEELS SPACED

Fluctuating consciousness
Evidence of organicity
Etiology
Learning and memory
Speech – incoherent
Sleep wake
Psychomotor – increased or decreased
Attention – decreased
Concentration – decreased
Experience hallucinations
Disorientation

DELUSIONAL DISORDER

NOAR

Non bizarre delusions
not **O**bviously bizarre behaviour
Auditory hallucinations, not prominent
Rule out affective, schizophrenia and organic

DEMENTIA

MAJOR PD

Memory loss – decreased short term and long term memory
Abstract thought decreased, Aphasia, Apraxia, Agnosia – four A's
Judgement decreased
Organicity presumed
Rule out depression and
Personality disorder
Decline in functioning at work and relationships

DEPRESSION

SIGE CAPS

Sleep disturbed
Interest diminished
Guilt
Energy decreased
Concentration decreased
Appetite and weight up or down
Psychomotor retardation or agitation
Suicidal

GENERALIZED ANXIETY DISORDER

STOMACH

Severity and vigilance
Two or more worries
Organic rule out
Motor tension
Anxiety unrelated
Course not psychotic
Hyper-reactive autonomic

HYPOCHONDRIASIS

FIND RS

Fear and preoccupation with disease
Interpret physical symptoms as evidence of illness
Normal on examination
Despite examination not reassured
Rule out panic disorder and psychosis
Six months

MANIA

GREAT SAD

Grandiose
Racing thoughts
Euphoria
Activities increased
Talkative
Sleep decreased, Sex increased
Activities self damaging and increased e.g. binge, spend, impulse
Distractible

OBSESSIVE COMPULSIVE DISORDER

RESIDENT PRISONER

Recurrent ideas
Experienced as
Senseless and attempt to
Ignore ideas
Drugs – rule out
Eating disorder – rule out
Not related to
Thought insertion – rule out

Purposeful
Repetitive
Intentional
Stereotyped
response to **O**bsession
Neutralisation
Excessive
interfere with **R**outine

PANIC ATTACK

DPIF

Discrete
Periods of
Intense
Fear

PANIC DISORDER

CATASTROFIES

Choking
Angina
Tachycardia
Abdominal distress
Sweat
Tremble
Rule out other anxiety disorders
Fear of dying or going crazy
Intense
Escape
SOB – short of breath

POST-TRAUMATIC STRESS DISORDER

DREAMS

Disinterest and detachment
Re-experience nightmares and flashbacks
Events, type or single trauma, multiple
Avoidance of the situations, thoughts that invoke trauma
Month – greater than one
Sympathetic hyperactivity, exaggerated startle response (*hypervigilance*)

PREMORBID PERSONALITY

HERMI

Habitual defences
Egoistic strength
Relationships
Mood stability
Impulsivity/identity

SCHIZOPHRENIA

ACID PH SODAS

Affect
Catatonia
Incoherent language or speech
Delusions
Prominent **H**allucinations
rule out **S**chizoaffective
rule out **O**rganic
Decline in functioning
Autism – consider
Six months

SOMATIZATION

PONSE

Physical complaints, no panic
Onset <30 years
No organicity
Symptoms – many
Effects, take medications

SUICIDE

SUICIDAL

S

Sex – female>male

Significant others – lonely, single, widowed, care for child, protective factor

Stressful life events – loss of loved one, finances, job loss

U

Unsuccessful attempts

Unemployment

Unexplained improvement (in clinical features – often result of deciding on a suicide plan)

I

Identification (with family members)

CI

Chronic illness – or severe illness of recent onset, increased risk of successful suicide

Depression and bipolar affective disorder and schizophrenia increase the risk

D

Depression, hopelessness, frustration, hostility – associated with risk

A

Age – increased age increases risk

Alcohol – increase risk, substance abuse

Availability of weapons, guns

L

Lethality of previous attempts, guns, hanging jumping from high places